AF657391

Patient-Physician Relationship

Patient-Physician Relationship

Edited by
Ratna Dutta Sharma
Sashinungla

Decent Books
New Delhi

in collaboration with

Department of Philosophy
Jadavpur University
Kolkata

Cataloging in Publication Data — DK
[Courtesy: D.K. Agencies (P) Ltd. <docinfo@dkagencies.com>]

Patient-physician relationship / edited by Ratna Dutta Sharma, Sashinungla.
xiii, 257 p.; 23 cm.
Most of the papers presented at the Workshop on Perspectives of the Patient-physician relationship, held at Calcutta.
Includes bibliograhical references.
Includes index.
ISBN 8186921419

1. Physician and patient — Congresses. 2. Physician and patient — India — Congresses. 3. Medical ethics — Congresses. I. Sharma, Ratna Dutta, 1952- II. Sashinungla, 1975-.

DDC 610.696 22

ISBN 81-86921-41-9
First Published in India in 2007
© Jadavpur University, Kolkata.

All rights reserved. No part of this publication may be reproduced or transmitted in any form or by any means, electronic or mechanical, including photocopying, recording or any information storage or retrieval system, without prior written permission of both the copyright owner, indicated above, and the publisher.

Published by:
Decent Books
D-36/A-1, Mohan Garden
Najafgarh Road
New Delhi - 110 059
Ph. (011) 2535-3435

in collaboration with

Department of Philosophy
Jadavpur University
Kolkata (West Bengal)

Distributed by:
D.K. Printworld (P) Ltd.
Regd. office : *'Sri Kunj,'* F-52, Bali Nagar
Ramesh Nagar Metro Station
New Delhi - 110 015
Phones : (011) 2545-3975, 2546-6019; *Fax* : (011) 2546-5926
E-mail : dkprintworld@vsnl.net
Web : www.dkprintworld.com

Printed by: Decent Books, New Delhi

A Note

Applied Philosophy is one major thrust area of research of the Department of Philosophy under its ASIHSS (UGC's Assistance for Strengthening of the Infrastructure of the Humanities to Social Sciences) programme. The Research Group working in this area aims to show the relevance and applicability which philosophy has in dealing with problems encountered in different domains of practical life. This in fact is the aim of Applied Philosophy which, as normally conceived, is concerned with the elaboration of theories purported to give guidance for understanding and handling problems in concrete situations. The members of the group have chosen to specifically focus on problems relating to three domains: Teaching, Medicine and Law.

These general remarks however do not shed much light on the nature and scope of Applied Philosophy. It is better to resort to examples of specific problems in any of the chosen domains with reference to which we may understand how philosophy can be applied.

In the field of "teaching," one such problem could be about the nature and ultimate goal of the prevalent system of teaching. Does the goal, which the system sets before the students, ask for their personal excellence, achievement and professional success only? "Yes, indeed," might be our instant reply expressing an assertive and a received view. Then, how else will our honest and laborious efforts full of sweat, blood and tears be rewarded? It is possible by academic and professional ascents only. Some of us may be displeased when we think what this sort of achievement might lead to? There may be immense psychological pressure, unrestrained competition and self-assertion in the mind of the achiever who flourishes in self-seclusion making him forget the values of care and concern for others.

Philosophers do not have a monopoly in making pronouncements about such matters. But they do have a distinctive role in (1) making us aware of the problems. We need to clarify, analyze and even revise conceptions which generate these problems (in this case the conception concerning the goal of teaching). (2) They are also required to discern and make explicit some other conceptions, assumptions, theories and values which seem to support that problem-generating conception. (The underlying conception or theory here seems to be a right-based individualistic theory of justice). (3) The philosophers' task includes furthermore a critical evaluation, especially about the normative viability of the contentious view cited as an example, and also a consideration of other rival positions. Their task is to initiate debates and assess arguments advanced by the debating parties. (4) Yet another task is engagement with methodological issues. What method is to be deployed by practitioners of other disciplines to construct theories? What can be the criteria of theory-choice by applying which the rival claims of competing theories can be adjudicated?

These are some of the ways in which philosophy can be applied to other domains also, including the two other fields which the project has chosen, viz. Medicine and Law. A medical practitioner could be made aware of certain problems. Philosophical debates could be centred around such problems in fields of specialization. Some of these problems may be about — Freedom over one's body; Identity of life; Social implications of various treatments; Doctor-Patient relationship, etc. In the field of Law, the problems which merit scrutiny may be — Relation between legal rights and moral rights; Relation between legal rights and political rights; Relation between justice, law and power; gender justice; etc.

The typical facets of philosophical activity — conceptual, theoretical, normative, logical and methodological — considered here, do not exhaust the role of Applied Philosophy. In fact the very idea of applying general abstract theories to concrete situations has been challenged by many thinkers. But that too would be an issue which merits philosophical scrutiny.

The department had organized a seminar on the theme: **Health, Ethics and Law,** in collaboration with the Institute of Development Studies; a workshop on Education for Personality Development and Value; and a workshop on Nature and Need of Sex-education in School.

A workshop was also held on the theme: **Perspectives of the Patient-Physician Relationship** which comes under the purview of *Medicine*, one of the three major areas on which the project of Applied Philosophy has chosen to focus. The present volume has evolved extra efforts to address conceptual, theoretical, ethical, cultural, legal and methodological issues pertaining to this specific theme which have been elaborated in the Editor's Introduction. It is a collection of papers written by eminent philosophers and thinkers representing other disciplines. Most of the papers were presented at the workshop.

Chhanda Gupta
Professor and Co-ordinator
Applied Philosophy Research Group
UGC — ASIHSS Programme
Department of Philosophy
Jadavpur University

Contents

Acknowledgement

The workshop from which this book has emerged was funded by the University Grants Commission (UGC) and Jadavpur University, Kolkata. We are grateful to them for their support.

Our students, particularly the ones who are studying for their Masters and M. Phil degrees, helped us by showing unqualified enthusiasm. We are thankful to our colleagues for their support.

Ratna Dutta Sharma & Sashinungla

Introduction

Ratna Dutta Sharma

THE title of the present anthology is self-explanatory. Focusing especially on this theme it intends to bring out philosophical presuppositions underlying it and philosophical implications following therefrom. Is there anyone who has not sought the help of a medical professional, being afflicted with such ailments which demand medical care? The physician in course of treating a patient and the patient receiving treatment from the physician, both enter into a relationship with one another.

In general this relationship remains harmonious. Occasionally, however, it takes a bad turn resulting in loss of mutual trust, volley of allegations being levied against each other and often resulting in violence. For the benefit of the society and betterment of the individual, a harmonious and a balanced relation between the physician and the patient is imperative. This justifies the selection of this theme as the area of investigation. Patient-Physician relationship is one of the most important inter-disciplinary areas of research. The aim of the present anthology is to generate interface among philosophers, physicians, legal experts and the researchers engaged in investigative research work in this or related areas which will result in a proper conceptual understanding of the issues along with recent development in the area. The eventual goal is to gain future direction to get optimum result in health care domain.

The health care seeker approaches a health care professional for medical assistance. The physician charges fees for the service he renders. But do the physicians regard themselves as performing the health care service just for a fee or there are other dimensions, which motivate them?

The present trend of consumerism may take the patient to be the consumer of health service. But the question is — can this seller-consumer model explain the patient-physician relationship? Instances of selfless and dedicated physicians rendering free medical service to the community are innumerable. In cases of emergency, physicians often render required service without caring for remuneration. The physician not only treats the patient, but he is also concerned about the feeling and emotional responses of the patient to illness. In the words of Caraka, "A good physician nurtures affection for his patients exactly like the mother, father, brother and kinds." If this is true, the physician as a human being cannot but enter into an emotional attachment with the patient. Provided there is some sort of emotional bonding between the physician and the patient, the question now arises whether the physician can remain free from prejudice?

In the present socio-economic scenario, the physician is required to maintain a certain norm of conduct and a standard form of professionalism. This may indirectly debar the physician from entering into intimacy with the patients. They are often supposed to maintain a professional distance for the sake of their profession. The question remains — how can the relationship between physicians and their patients be both of the peculiar mixture — of detachment and involvement at the same time?

There are differences of opinion in regard to the nature of patient-physician relationship. The fact that the physician renders immense service to the health care seeker remains undisputed. But what role does the patient play in this matter? Are they mere recipients of the service provided by the physician or do they have any active role? According to some, the patient lacking the required expert knowledge depends on the physician for his medical care. The patients are also happy to leave everything to the physician who is always ready to act in the patient's best interests without his knowledge or consent.

This surely shows that the patient has trust and faith in the physician, which prompts him to follow the advice of the health care professionals. The trust and faith entrusted to the physician depends, to a large extent, on the belief that physicians are guided by the code of confidentiality. The obligation of confidentiality prohibits the physician from disclosing information about the patient's case to others and encourages him to take precaution with the information. But do the physicians believe in the utilitarian justification for confidentiality as stated above, or do they rely on the deontological arguments defending confidentiality? Deontological justification is based on the notions such as privacy, autonomy, promise-keeping, etc. But how far is the confidentiality to be maintained?

What additional factors are there which promote patient's adherence? This question is very important. Because most medical interventions rely on patient's adherence.

There has been a shift from the position holding "The physician knows the best" to a position where much greater emphasis is put on the patient's preference for the type of treatment desired. The former model may be discarded on the argument demanding patient's autonomy to be considered as a basic value. As a person the patient has the right to be informed of his own condition and to take his own decision on treatment. The patients must be provided with information regarding alternative methods of treatment and the risks involved therein to enable them to make a rational and intelligent choice. But the problem remains as to what extent the patient is to be informed? Should the patient be informed about the mistakes, if there be any, in diagnosis and management? Will the attempt to hide such mistakes amount to the violation of truth-telling?

Though communication plays an important role in patient-physician relationship, the problem associated with it can in no way be ignored. Is it possible for the patient to grasp the technical details of his disease and treatment? How to ascertain that the patient truly comprehends the information conveyed to him? One additional problem of the physician-patient communication is caused by the varied use of the concept of "health," "illness," "disease," etc. It is not unlikely that all these concepts represent distinct realities rather than shared realities. It is obvious that the physician should not respect all choices made by the patients. But he should respect the choice of a competent patient. But how to assess that the patient is competent enough to give his opinion in regard to the method of his treatment? If higher good, according to the patient, prevails, the patient may refuse to follow the physician's instructions in spite of being fully aware of the fact that this might lead to the sacrifice of what is biomedically good for him. Can the patient, in that case, be abandoned to his autonomy? What should the physician do if there is a conflict between the physician's obligations to do what he thinks would serve the best interest of the patient and his obligation to respect the patient's choice? A patient, suffering from head injuries and internal bleeding, for instance, may refuse the doctor's recommended blood transfusion because of his strong religious belief even though he is aware of the consequences of his refusal. Should the physician in that situation respect the patient's choice though he knows for certain that it would go against the best interest of the patient. The example mentioned above indicates the role that religion plays in determining patient-physician relationship. Can children and mentally ill patients give their opinion regarding their treatment method? The above discussion shows that there are a number of important problems associated with the different alternative ways of conceiving patient-physician relationship. Does it entail the necessity for actively exploring and experimenting with new ways of seeing and re-modelling this relationship?

Does the physician subject himself to the conviction that his relation with the patient should be commensurate with the nature and stage of the patient's ailment *vis-à-vis* its complications? What should be the relation of the physician with the terminally ill patient?

It is also an aspect to be dwelt upon that the physician-patient relationship varies depending on the different branches of medical treatment being adapted.

How far cultural factors contribute to this relationship, can be apprehended by an example. Judaism, for instance, considers that Jewish prayer is a powerful healing tool as well as an integral part of patient care.

Do the medical professionals need to have different ways of dealing with male and female patients? We may refer to the news published in the *Hindustan Times* on 14 December, 2005. This, I presume, would suggest the direction of the answer. The male doctors in Orissa want a number of safeguards to be put in place before they treat women patients. The arrest and suspension of some doctors on charge of sexual exploitation of women patients have unnerved them to such an extent that they are reluctant to examine women patients even in government hospitals in the absence of female attendants or nurses. This reminds us of Caraka's instruction to the physicians not to attend a lady in the absence of her husband or guardian.

Individual characteristics of doctors and patients, to a certain extent, definitely affect how they relate to each other. Such attributes include personal values, attitudes and beliefs. For instance, a physician A has the reputation of being very competent and very friendly with his patients, gives an advance appointment over the telephone. Another physician B, residing in the same locality of A, is also very competent but is too commercial. He treats his patients as objects and things and not as persons. Naturally a patient P would feel comfortable to consult A and not B.

If there are so many determinants of physician-patient relationship, then this would vary accordingly depending on the diverse factors. In that case the question would be — is there anything common among these diverse possibilities?

Both the physician and the patient contribute to this relationship which is of utmost importance for medical treatment. We find in *Caraka Saṁhitā,* Caraka has specified what a physician should and should not do. He has further stipulated the qualities to be possessed by a patient for the achievement of optimum result.

The Medical Council of India Notification, dated 11 March, 2002 has specified the duties and responsibilities of the physicians. There is a legal guideline also for the duties to be discharged by the physician. But do the laws of India provide any duty for the physician? Yes, the Supreme Court held that the duty of the physician includes:

a. a duty of care in deciding whether to undertake a case;

b. a duty of care in deciding what treatment to give; and

c. a duty of care in administration of that treatment.

Regarding the first stipulated duty, it may be asked what are the specific grounds on which the physician may refuse to undertake a case.

What does the expression "duty of care" actually mean? How far the right of a patient to participate in the decision-making of his treatment exists in reality in medical practice?

Does any breach of duty on the part of the physician make him liable for any offence?

Is it possible for the patient to take any legal step against a physician if he fails to discharge his allotted duties?

The Supreme Court of India in its landmark judgement laid down the law relating to professional negligence under Consumer Protection Act, 1986. Does it not necessarily assume the patient to be a "consumer"? But in what particular sense a patient can be taken to be a consumer? It was held that the relationship that holds between a physician and a patient could be treated as a contract of service. But does the word "contract" convey any special significance?

Now the question arises — do the patients really have the capacity to fight back? Because the Consumer Court requires two doctors to verify that the case has merit before accepting a complaint against the doctor. But actually doctors refuse to opine against another doctor.

What constitutes gross act of negligence on the part of the physician? Does the mere lack of necessary care, attention and skill of the physician amount to gross negligence?

All these show that the focus on the patient-physician relationship brings us to such fields as law and philosophy of law also. Apart from the above, there are a number of other areas that should be dealt with and discussed for doing justice to the specific topic. But it is not possible to focus on all the relevant areas at the same time. For this reason we have decided to be confined to the areas which are relevant to understand the crux of the patient-physician relationship.

The contributors are experts in their respective fields. All of them have discussed in detail the various issues related to patient-physician relationship.

Debashis Chatterjee in his paper titled *Doctor-Patient Relationship: Nature and Boundaries,* suggests that our task is to look into the components and vicissitudes that occur in relationship to influence the outcome. He has also made an attempt to find out the conditions which are responsible for bringing a major paradigm shift in the relation. The different crucial components of all doctor-patient relationship have been analyzed. The fundamental tenets on which the ethics of medical profession have been based, is also pointed out with due emphasis.

Pushpa Misra in her paper titled *Patient-Physician Relationship: Ethical Perspectives,* has concentrated on the ethical dimensions of a patient-physician relationship. The first section of the paper deals with the principles of medical ethics. The second section has been devoted to the consideration of the medical conditions prevailing in the state of West Bengal with respect to the above-mentioned ethical principles. The purpose is to highlight the influence of the social and cultural factors influencing patient-physician relationship. In the third section of the paper, she has stipulated what she considers to be the best approach in medical ethics.

Amit Kumar Sharma in his paper *Culture as Determinant of Patient-Physician Relationship in Ayurveda,* has tried to point out the role that culture plays as a guiding force to a *vaidya* while dealing with his/her patient. He has considered the different important dimensions of patient-physician relationship.

S.Y. Khan, after clarifying the concept of "relationship," "religion" and "Islam," has tried to find out the *Role of Religion (Islam) and Sex as Determinant of Patient-Physician Relationship.* He has concentrated on some specific contexts of serious illness that dive into the realm of religion. Khan has specifically elaborated some of the situations, namely — confrontation with self-mortality, coping with affliction and the desire for companionship.

Swaraj Mazumdar in the first part of his paper *Patient-Physician Relationship: A Homoeopath's Appraisal* has tried to show that homoeopathy is not faith healing. It is a perfect, holistic healing art as well as a science. He has also attempted to show how a homoeopath treats his patients and what are the advantages of such a treatment over other methods with special reference to patient-doctor relationship and cost-effectiveness. The second part deals with problems that a homoeopath has to face in treating his patients and developing a relationship based on mutual trust and confidence. The author has concluded that a Vedāntic approach, which is the basis of all ethical values, is very important if we want to cast the physician-patient relationship in a new mould.

Sashinungla explores a particular tribal tradition, namely the Aos of Nagaland in the light of contemporary understanding of what is believed as indigenous medicine. Her paper *Indigenous Concept of Medicine* holds that indigenous Ao medicine is a holistic healing approach that emphasizes the treatment of body, mind, and spirit. The spiritual rejuvenation and the achievement of a general sense of physical, emotional, and communal harmony, she points out, are at the heart of indigenous Ao medicine. The paper discusses the methods, reputation and performance of the indigenous healer-patient relationship. She claims that the indigenous Ao healer's role stands at the interstices of religion, spiritism and social system and gains its power from this position. Sashi also points out the need to address critical issues like imposition of epistemological foundations of western knowledge on indigenous knowledge systems with the result that the biological and intellectual tradition of non-western understanding was devalued.

The title of the paper *Caraka and the Notification of the Indian Medical Council, on Patient-Physician Relationship* by Ratna Dutta Sharma is self-explanatory. In this paper she has tried to make a comparative study. Caraka has dealt with every important aspect of this relation. On different points the position of Caraka have been maintained even in the recent Declaration of the Indian Medical Council 2002 with required modifications. Some of the views of Caraka have been dropped in the recent notification. The reason for all these changes, according to the author, can be traced back mainly to the changed social conditions.

In the paper *Non-Reason, Madness, Mental Health Science and the "Ethics of Psychoanalysis"* Anup Kumar Dhar & Ranjita Biswas have raised different relevant questions — Does "unreason" get reduced to "madness" in the epistemic institution of "mental health science?" Does the institution of mental health science only rein in the "mind?" Does it not try to understand the "mind?" Does it attend to the complex vicissitudes of the "mind" only through abstract "Reason?" Does it attend to "unreason" only through "Reason?" Do certain moments in the large canvas of "mental health science" attend to "unreason?" Are these moments — moments that turn to "unreason" — related in ways more than one to psychoanalysis? Can psychoanalysis set up a meaningful engagement with unreason and not reduce it to mere madness? How one could still think of a possible relationship with unreason that could be ethical not just at the level of institutional practice but even at the level of knowledge/truth production?

Somdatta Bhattacharyya in her paper has focused on the concept of confidentiality, which is of utmost importance specifically for the relation of a patient to a physician who is concerned with the mental health of the former. In fact if the patient is not sure that the information which he or she has communicated to the therapist will remain confidential, the treatment cannot even proceed. If such confidential information is divulged, then the physician-client relationship may face some serious problems. The author has referred to such problems and their possible solution. She has raised some questions, which according to her, need the attention of the philosophers.

1. Is deliberate concealment of truth necessarily dishonest?
2. Is lying for the benefit of the patient a betrayal of trust?
3. How should therapists resolve conflict between their duty to be truthful and their other duties?

The evolution of consent in medical parlance is a recent event in comparison to the Hippocratic oath, nurtured by the ongoing changes in the perception of disease. This has been brought on by newer scientific advancements in the diagnosis and treatment of hitherto irremediable illnesses and the discovery of new disease agents and their manifestations. A challenge is posed by the increasing burden of expectations closing in on the traditional model of the all-powerful doctor pitted against a hapless patient. In a rapidly shrinking world where communication and transfer of information occur instantly, heightened knowledge and awareness of the health care seeker have shifted the balance of power to a more even ground of mutual concordance.

Nandini Banerjee, in her paper *A Glimpse into the Domain of Consent in the Doctor-Patient Relationship — Is it a Myth or Reality?* has looked into the evolution of the doctrine of consent taking into consideration the ethical principles governing it and also the professional and legal guidelines existing on this subject. It goes on to discuss what consent is all about by reflecting upon the problems commonly encountered in day-to-day clinical practice weighing the pros and cons and working its way around to find solutions to these dilemmas. In conclusion, it reiterates the fact that medicine lies in the interface of science and art and what appears merely to be a study of ill health or infirmity of the human organism is in reality a study of its mind and soul.

Patient-Physician Relationship for Conducting a Clinical Trial: A Look on Ethical Aspects and Role of Statistical Designs, by Gopaldeb Chattopadhyay, has concentrated on bio-ethics in the context of patient-physician relationship and the role of statistical methodologies for conducting a more ethical clinical trial especially on human subjects. The increased sensitivity to ethical issues generates a desire to conduct clinical trials, which are more ethical. At the same time there are advances in statistical thinking, computation facilities are also expanding resulting in capability of doing things differently, patients are becoming better informed, social contexts are changing. The author believes that the interplay of these changes forces us to think alternatively.

Malay Kumar Basu in his paper *Medicine and Law — In Perspective of Physician-Patient Relationship,* has emphasized that the laws on medicine in the perspective of doctor-patient relationship owe their origin and development to the changing needs of the society throughout the different ages since time immemorial. He has enumerated some of the major statutes in the chronological order which were enacted by our legislature from time to time for regulating the medical profession by spelling out the criteria of reasonable care and competence and standard of professional knowledge and skill and the various duties of a doctor. He has referred to a few landmark judgements touching on the significance of the physician-patient relations and the different factors contributing to it. Basu has suggested that as in all other spheres of life, revival of the ethical values and imparting of moral education can bring about a healthy relation between the patient and the physician.

The paper titled *Status of Patient and Physicians in Indian Scenario and its Improvement for Delivery of Better Healthcare* by Bansi Badan Mukhopadhyay concerned with the function and improvement of hospital services as well as the improvement of other health care centres. The author has emphasized that an attempt is to be made to improve the quality of services directed towards the role of patients, physician and management for providing better health care. As in most of the cases patients seeking care in government hospitals are illiterate and ignorant of their rights, he points out that the patients need to be educated and enlightened to enable them to exercise their rights.

Shefali Moitra in her paper *Some Feminist Concerns About Medical Practice* has shown that a great injustice is being done to women in regard to various aspects of their health related matters. Except the women reproductive functions and their malfunctioning all other women related complaints are treated by general medicine. But it is not proper to treat without reference to the gender difference of an individual. The attention has been given to research and development relating to women's reproductive health only. This, according to the author, is solely due to the fact that patriarchy emphasizes on the role, which a woman is, expected to perform as women. There is no doubt that sometimes the attempts, which the women take for the fulfilment of these expectations, are detrimental to their health. The research works in relation to women reproductive health has little to do with women's reproductive rights. The attitude towards women's body and its ailments demands drastic change. The method of diagnosis needs to be re-examined. The deplorable state of women's health, especially in the third world countries, according to the author is not only due to the negligence of State and family but also to the attitude of the women towards themselves, which the author believes to be the consequences of the internalization of the mindset of patriarchy as responsible for this. The author has given due emphasis on the implementation of the proposal given at the International Conference on Population and Development held in Cairo in 1994 for the improvement of the situation.

1

Doctor-Patient Relationship
Nature and Boundaries

Debashis Chatterjee

MEDICINE is supposed to be one of the oldest professions. From time immemorial doctors are trying to relieve pain and distress in others (albeit against financial compensations). But the history of predictable intervention strategies does not date back to more than two hundred years. So what were doctors doing all these years? Just calling them frauds and charlatans does not really answer the question because "getting better" is/was a real experience. Otherwise the profession would not have survived.

It is our belief that doctor-patient relationship was the effective tool that brought about changes in the person in pain. The relationship in itself carries the potential to bring in some desirable change in the ailing help-seeker. Our task is to look into the components and vicissitudes that occur in this relationship to influence the outcome.

The profession of medicine started in shamanism and magical practices. Even today the profession carries a strong streak of those beliefs and practices. This is not to say that these are anachronisms or bad but they can bring out the true nature of doctor-patient relationship.

The necessary myth in any kind of medical intervention is a belief that "knowledge" brings out some kind of betterment over "ignorance." Throughout the history of human civilization this duality of "knowledge-ignorance" has been allegorized as the duality between "light-dark." The tradition of medicine carries a strong echo of the same. Having technical information gives rise to a better "understanding" of a given situation. And correct utilization/manipulation of this technical information brings in a change/"improvement" in a given undesirable condition. Freudian psychotherapy is fundamentally based on the belief that if I "really" know what is wrong with me, the "wrong" shall disappear. Information-sharing is a large component to doctor-patient relationship and having acquired information tends to enhance the autonomy of the patient.

In many shamanic practices, the patient was not disturbed in anyway but the doctor used to imitate the ailments. It was a practice of homoeopathic magic (borrowing terms from James Frazer) that was believed to take away the pain from the patient as if the doctor, by imitating the patient's condition, could take the pain away from the patient onto his own body. When John Christian Reil, about two hundred years back, first coined the term "psychiatry," he used the word psyche in exactly this sense, that is using the doctor's psyche to find help for the patient (unfortunately, over the years, "psychiatry" has come to mean the patient's psyche). The use of empathy in today's psychotherapy employs the same general principle.

The last two centuries have witnessed two important paradigm shifts in doctor-patient relationship. In the small rural agrarian community a doctor was always a well-known local person, almost a family member. Quite frequently he took a paternal role for the individual and also for the family. He used to get invitations for family functions, was consulted for various family matters apart from medical problems like local politics, daughter's marriage, etc. On all such subjects he was himself free in dispensing his "learned" advice and sharing his experience.

Consequently there was a high level of trust in the relationship and a proportionate lack of autonomy. In fact in the then world, autonomy was not a primary concern of citizenship.

Industrialization and urbanization have brought in a major paradigm shift in this relation. Doctor now is just another faceless, anonymous citizen who has specific technical expertise (defined by acquisition of state-approved qualifications), whom you find and choose depending on the information available to you and who is supposed to help you gain specific changes in your body/mind conditions. Obviously, the outcome is a relatively low level of trust and high degree of autonomy on the client's part.

The second paradigm shift derives directly from the first, the lessening of "do good"-ism and enhancement of autonomy of patient in doctor-patient relationship. This has occurred in parallel of the changing views and ideas in modern social thoughts and citizenship ideals.

Components

All individual doctor-patient relationships are built on two components. They are the reality-based and the fantasy-based components.

The reality-based component, the *therapeutic alliance,* is basically a contract — on the part of the doctor to engage his best technical expertise for the patients's good and on the patient's part to respect the financial agreement and practical arrangements of appointment, etc. There is also an unwritten agreement that the patient will follow the doctor's advice or at least engage in discussion if she/he finds the advices difficult/unacceptable.

A doctor is supposed to bring to the relationship her/his technical knowledge, expertise and empathy and nothing else, especially no personal views and idiosyncrasies. On the other hand the patient brings to the relationship her/his views, beliefs and expectations and ingrained habits. These beliefs and expectations are largely formed by the patient's past life-experiences, which she/he tends to put on the doctor. This in turn tends to impair the doctor's "objectivity" and provokes his personal life-experience. This is the play of *transference — counter-transference* that is largely fantasy-based and forms a crucial component of all doctor-patient relationships.

Thus the process of doctor-patient relationship goes through the following steps: assessment and evaluation, rapport building, therapeutic alliance, transference and of course specific techniques (e.g. surgery) if and when indicated.

Placebo

The healing component of a doctor-patient relationship (accounting for 20-30% of therapeutic outcome) is often termed placebo or placebo effect. This term is problematic in the sense that we know placebo "effects" but we don't know how, and the magnitude of effect is not predictable. Thus frequently the term comes to mean a deception, which is neither true nor desirable. "Non-specific effect" has been offered as an alternative but we now know that some pain-placebo utilizes the specific analgesic neural pathways. "Expectation effect" may be a better alternative because placebo seriously depends on patient's expectations, both conscious and unconscious. The prognostic factors that determine the placebo outcome are explanatory models, sharing, ventilation acceptance, hope generation and magical expectancy. Knowledge imparted also plays a crucial role especially in promoting patient autonomy.

Definitions

Before proceeding let us review a few accepted definitions:

Health implies the relative absence of pain and discomfort and a continuous adaptation and adjustment to the environment to ensure optimal function.

Disease implies physio/psychological dysfunction.

Illness is the subjective state of distress.

Sickness is the social role adopted due to illness.

These are the definitions of medical literature. The concepts are not expected to be clear in a patient's mind and each of these carries an explanatory story with it. It is important to hit a point of congruency between the patient's explanatory "story" and to the doctor's explanatory "model" for the therapeutic process to progress.

Problems

To place doctor-patient relationship *vis-à-vis* today's changing social milieu, brings out a lot of problem points some of which seem to be unanswerable at the present juncture.

Who is a Doctor? In all "civilized" states today medical curriculum is state-sponsored/supervised. This seems to be a must if a minimum standard of training is to be maintained, but this, on the other hand, tends to put a lot of abusable power in the state's hand. Can a doctor be self-proclaimed in today's world? The other question is whether different system doctors like allopaths (whatever be the meaning of the term), homoeopaths, kaviraji and unani practitioners all will be bound by the same category of doctor-patient relationships and ethical guidelines.

Violence: Modern medicine is vivisectionist and reductionist. These seem to be irretrievably woven into the basic philosophy of medical science. Even small intervention strategies like parenteral routes of drug delivery, surgical techniques, etc. bring out a natural picture of violence in the mind of the help-seeker and acts as a deterrent from the very act of help-seeking. A medical practitioner conjures up a picture of a violent person and at least the near future does not seem to offer any change in this.

Congruency of Explanatory Models: This is one area where quite frequently a practitioner in modern medicine flounders in dealing with real patients especially in areas of psychological dysfunction. In our community, a common occurrence is a young man presenting with psycho-physiological problems that he believes are due to "loss of semen." Now, in Bengali semen is *"dhātu"* which also means metal or base material. Thus, loss of semen carries for him a plethora of culturally relevant significance like, loss of "life-essence," manliness, courage, vitality ad infinitum. In medical terminology, loss of semen in non-understable/non-significant models commonly used by a doctor like "depression" or "anxiety" in turn carries little significance to the help-seeker. This lack of congruency invariably leads to breakdown of the therapeutic relationship and leaves the patient in the lurch. Another common example is the case of so-called "possession syndrome." A similar lack of congruency occurs there.

Doctor as an Agent: Therapeutic contract, like any other contract in civil society, presupposes free agency for the contract makers. In the therapeutic contract the patient is always, by definition, free but the doctor may not be so. His obligations to his employer may come into conflict with the best interests of the patients. A common example is a doctor employed in her/his country's armed forces. A related but graver problem is because in today's society the state is the provider/arbiter for medical curriculum, the state may choose to claim doctors as its agents if and when a conflict between state interest and citizens' interest arises. History of twentieth century medical practice brings out innumerable situations where doctors willingly or unwillingly collude with state power against the interest of the citizens. Another problem is the case of third party payment. When an insurance company mediates between a doctor and a patient, it tends to undermine the autonomy of both. Doctor-patient unethical collusion to deceive the third party (i.e. insurance company) is also a real threat, even to an honest doctor-patient relationship.

Two Faces of Doctor-Patient Relationship: Medical science, as a branch of science in general, is supposed to be objective and impersonal. In a doctor-patient relationship the doctor is the distant "knower," an impersonal collector and dispenser of information while the patient is the distanced knowable/known subject. But the therapeutic relation does not go that way. Here a doctor has to be a non-judgemental acceptor of the personality of the patient and has to extend warm regard for the patient. All practitioners of medicine have to learn this inherent and often insurmountable duality and contradiction in her/his professional career.

Ethics

Ethical considerations lay the ground for all successful doctor-patient relationships but here too a lot of questions are unanswered.

Codified ethics or law depends on implementing agency and mechanisms of implementation. Unfortunately, till date, both remain largely non-functional and our society seems to be as yet uncertain as to how to deal with the issue. Laws are there in galore but utilization and implementation remains a problem.

Introduction of managed care in big insured private hospitals bring in its own problems like erosion of confidentiality, decreased autonomy of patients, split treatment module and shrinkage in types of reimbursable services.

Ethics of medical practices depends upon the following basic tenets: Beneficence, Non-malfeasance, Autonomy, Justice, Confidentiality and Veracity. The first two involve the competence of the care-giver and in turn depend on the individual's capacity and idiosyncrasies and the quality of the training curriculum, which is often determined by the state. Relative importance and primacy of the different tenets have varied over time and in different societies. As said earlier, till about two hundred years back, beneficence and non-malfeasance were most important. The Hippocratic oath first formulated this ground rule. Margaret Mead pointed out that this was the first time in history that power to heal and power to kill were separated and doctors as a professional community were directed to practise the first and were barred from practising the second. She also pointed out that with Hippocratic oath emerged the concept of virtue as a compensation/reward for professional ethical conduct. Coming of modern civic society shifted the primacy from beneficence to autonomy, and evolving post-modern society seems again to change it to justice and veracity.

Concept of boundary in doctor-patient relationship involves not only the patient's interest but third party interest as well. The doctor is supposed to be responsible not only to his individual client but to society in general. This dual obligation may often lead to ethical dilemmas and doctor's agencyhood may come into question.

MEDICINE: PROFESSION OR TRADE?

In 1975 the USA Supreme Court rendered a decision, Goldfarb vs. Virginia State Bar Association that changed the way professions were to be considered and regulated. The verdict ended the "learned professions exemption" under the Sherman Antitrust Act. Goldfarb, an attorney himself, sued the Virginia Bar Association because he found that all attorneys in Fairfax County, where he wanted to buy a house, were charging the same fees to conduct a title search. He contended that this was restraint of trade, and the Supreme Court agreed with him. Not long after the Goldfarb decision was announced, the Federal Trade Commission (FTC) of USA sued American Medical Association holding that the AMA was in restraint of trade because its codes of ethics prohibited advertising. USA Supreme Court decided the case in 1982 in favour of FTC. Medicine in effect ceased to be a profession — at least in the traditional sense of an autonomous association self-regulated by a code of ethics — and became a trade.

Though this happened in far off USA, it deeply involves us all in today's globalized (read Americanized) world. If medicine becomes a trade, the whole of doctor-patient relationship and medical ethics will require a new look and thorough rewriting.

2

Doctor-Patient Relationship
Ethical Principles vs. Socio-Cultural Factors

Pushpa Misra

IN this paper, I will discuss the ethical dimensions of a doctor-patient relationship. This paper is divided into three sections. In the first section, I will discuss the principles of medical ethics. The second section will give some details of the medical conditions prevailing in the state of West Bengal with respect to these ethical principles. This will highlight the influence of the social and cultural factors in the doctor-patient relationship. In the third and final section, I will try to sketch an argument to establish why a judicious combination of the principle of beneficence and autonomy is the best approach in medical ethics.

I

What is Medical Ethics?

Ethics is the science of rightness and wrongness of human conduct. In its most familiar sense when we talk about morality with reference to human conduct we have in mind a set of norms that govern human conduct in general.

Medical ethics is a set of norms by which the rightness and wrongness of the people belonging to medical profession is guided and evaluated. Thus, medical ethics is a form of professional morality. Every profession has its specific moral requirements that are related to the special nature of that profession. When we enter into a professional relationship with anyone we enter into a formal or informal contract to receive certain services in exchange of certain obligations on our part. Medical profession is probably the most important of all professions because when x enters into a medical relation with y (y may be a physician or a medical institution), x entrusts her most valuable treasure, namely her life and health, into the hands of y. It is, therefore, not without reason that the need for a stringent moral norm was felt for the medical profession. "In medicine professional morality specifies general moral norms for the institutions, practices, and traditions of medicines." — (*Principles of Biomedical Ethics* — Beauchamp and Childress, p. 5).

Like all professions, medical profession was also initially guided by certain informal moral norms. In Western tradition, we are familiar with Hippocratic oath which the fresh medical graduates are still required to take. In Indian tradition, Maharṣi Caraka had given very specific moral norms that were supposed to guide the doctor's duties *vis-à-vis* his patients.[1] These principles were transmitted from the teacher to the disciple and were carried on from one generation to another. It is quite natural that in this process of oral transmission the original form and content of these principles will undergo significant changes. The Hippocratic oath dates back to fourth century BCE. It had two basic parts. The first part deals with the duties of the physician towards his teacher. For example, he should treat his teacher as his parent; he should teach the son/sons of his teacher without taking any fee, the physician

1. See Dr. Ratna Sen Sharma.

is obliged to pass on his knowledge to the next generation because the knowledge is God-given and he should always consider himself as being in debt for being given this knowledge. The second part of the oath deals with the truly ethical codes that determine the duties of the doctor towards his patients. They deal with such topics as confidentiality, refraining from sexual contact with the patient, to be sensitive to the sufferings of the patient, and above all the famous rule *Primus non nocere* — "First, do no harm to the patient." The Declaration of Geneva — the modern version of Hippocratic oath known as the neo-Hippocratic oath — retained the last mentioned rule in its place of honour.

Beginning of modern medical ethics dates back to 1960s. After immense discussions, philosophers have agreed upon four principles which will guide the behaviour and duties of the physician towards his patients. These principles are:

1. Respect for autonomy of the patient
2. Non-maleficence
3. Beneficence
4. Justice

It is to be noted that these are abstract principles. Specific rules and duties are to be derived by applying these principles in concrete situations. Adherence to these principles in solving moral dilemmas and in determining the duties of the physician is called principlism. It should, however, be noted that in case of conflict between principles an absence of hierarchy makes it difficult to resolve the conflict.

RESPECT FOR AUTONOMY OF THE PATIENT

The word "autonomy" has a Greek origin — *'auto'* means self and *'nomos'* means rules or laws. So, it is used to mean "self-rule" normally in case of self-governance of independent city-states. The principle here, however, is applied to mean personal autonomy. In their classic text *Principles of Biomedical Ethics*, Beauchamp and Childress say —

> To respect an autonomous agent is, at a minimum, to acknowledge that person's right to hold views, to make choices, and to take actions based on personal values and beliefs. Such action involves respectful *action*, not merely a respectful *attitude* . . . Respect, on this account, involves acknowledging decision-making rights and enabling persons to act autonomously, whereas disrespect for autonomy involves attitudes and actions that ignore, insult, or demean others' rights of autonomy. — (*Principles of Biomedical Ethics* — Beauchamp and Childress).

The essential component of personal autonomy is freedom from both external and internal control. In decision-making one needs to have adequate information as well as the capacity to understand. Mentally retarded persons cannot be considered as having full autonomy because of limited intellectual capacity, but having this capacity alone does not guarantee autonomous decision in the absence of all relevant information.

The philosophical basis of respect for autonomy comes from Kant's two maxims: "Always treat a person as an end and never merely as a means." His other maxim — "Every person is a member of the Kingdom of Ends," also lends support to the principle of autonomy.

An autonomous person is a rational agent, a moral agent "free and capable of making decisions."

Applied to doctor-patient relationship, respect for autonomy has the following practical implications:

i. A Patient has Right to informed consent;

ii. A Patient has Right to medical confidentiality; and

iii. A Patient has Right to know the truth about her illness.

Informed consent

It was only after 1970 that the term "informed consent" came into vogue. The Nuremburg trial and the associated Nazi atrocities made the medical world aware of the need of the consent of the patient in the medical procedure to be applied on her. However, the concept has not been a very clear one, and its application in the practical field has often been quite difficult due to factors we will discuss shortly. According to Beauchamp and Childress, the following elements are involved in any informed consent:

(IC1) Competence to understand and decide

(IC2) Disclosure

(IC3) Recommendation of a plan

(IC4) Understanding

(IC5) Voluntariness

(IC6) Decision

(IC7) Authorization.

All the above factors have remained highly debatable within the medical fraternity.

(IC1) to (IC7) require the following:

The patient is to be honestly given all the information necessary for arriving at a decision. They should be given not only all the alternative plans of treatment available, but the physician should also recommend a specific plan to the patient. This will give the patient an idea of what the physician thinks most important in making a decision. It is important that the patient is intellectually and emotionally competent to understand the information given to them. This involves that the patient has understood her diagnosis, prognosis, the nature of medical intervention, the risks and benefits involved in the intervention and the recommended plan of the physician. It is also important that the patient has made the decision free from pressure whether external or internal. Chemical dependency, psychiatric disorder or a debilitating disease might create internal pressure in favour of a particular medical intervention. When these requirements are satisfied, it is only then that the physician is properly authorized to perform the proposed medical intervention.

Each of these above seven factors brings enormous difficulties when we come to apply them in the practical field. Competence has always remained a controversial factor especially in the field of psychiatric medicine. Consider the following case:

Mrs A is an intelligent, well-educated lady, separated from her husband. She has been hospitalized with a diagnosis of schizoaffective disorder. Mrs A is a very competent lady. After she improved, she had been assigned and performed very efficiently a host of jobs in the hospital as part of her occupational therapy. She, however, has quite a bit of megalomanic tendencies, thinks everyone else as her inferior and incompetent compared to her. She also has a network of delusional belief about her husband which, however, does not affect her day-to-day functioning. She suffers from bouts of depression which she assigns to the hospital atmosphere. She is very unhappy with the atmosphere of the hospital and wants to live by herself.

Can Mrs A be considered competent to take decision about her life? She does have superior intellectual abilities and her delusions did not interfere with her everyday activities. Yet can the physicians treating her take the risk of allowing her to live alone and entrust the psychiatric medicine to be kept with her? She suffers from bouts of depression and because of her megalomanic tendencies is very difficult to get along with. Yet she is capable of performing the normal daily activities. How competent one has to be in order to be considered competent?

In addition to the ambiguity involved in the concept of "competence" there are at least three major difficulties related to informed consent.

(D1) — Some physicians point out that very often the knowledge base of the patient to understand the nature of disease is very inadequate. Lack of this knowledge also interferes with their proper understanding of the exact nature of medical intervention . . .

> . . . Simply, no non-medical professional can reasonably be expected to understand the details of the medical procedure. So basing the requirement for consent upon a requirement that the patient understands, those details would make consent almost impossible to obtain. — (*The Cambridge Medical Ethics Workbook* — Michael Parker and Donna Dickenson).

(D2) — There may be difficulties related to information processing — what the doctor has said and what the patient has understood may often differ widely. Information processing also depends on whether the information has been presented in positive or negative language. For example, the physician saying that there is 40% chance of survival presents a different picture compared to his saying that there is 60% chance of not surviving the procedure.

(**D3**) — There are important social difficulties that hinder proper understanding. These difficulties are embedded in the specific social factors. For example, the patient might not understand that they are free not to give their consent, or that they are free to take a second opinion. Such distortions are often embedded in the social structure and sometimes in the micro-situation of the patients themselves.

One of the very important questions is: How far the respect for autonomy should be stretched? Should the physician allow the patient to commit suicide? Should he feel obliged to accept the decision of the patient even if his medical knowledge says that the intervention will be harmful for the patient? The case of Peter Knoll has become the focus of controversy in this respect.

Peter Knoll — a 56 year old Swiss law professor was diagnosed with advanced cancer of the bladder. Surgery combined with radiation usually gives fairly good chances of survival though the lifestyle becomes restricted. Sexual intercourse will not be possible for him after surgery and he would have to carry a urine collecting bag. Peter refused treatment. His surgeon said that he had great respect for his decision but requested him to take a second opinion. Peter did not. As Peter Knoll said in his book *In the face of Death*:

> What bothers me is the loss of freedom, having others in charge of you, to be drawn into a medical machine which controls a person and which one cannot fight. Naturally, intolerable pain will disturb me too. In order to escape it, one enters the machine that takes away pain and at the same time freedom. And it's precisely this enslavement that I don't want. (*The Cambridge Medical Ethics Workbook* — Parker, Michael and Dickenson Donna, p. 271).

Peter Knoll died one year after the diagnosis. True to his spirit of independence he lived alone and even administered his own pain-relieving medicines. He continued to write till the last day and planned his own funeral.

Confidentiality: Confidentiality is also an old rule of ethics and has been mentioned in the Hippocratic oath.

The World Medical Association's Declaration of Geneva asserts an obligation of "absolute secrecy" and includes the following pledge: "I will respect the secrets which are confided in me, even after the patient dies." — (*Principle of Biomedical Ethics* — Beauchamp and Childress, 2001, p. 304).

Confidentiality is related to a person's right to privacy. When information that has been imparted on the basis of trust are disclosed to a third party without the permission of the informant, an infringement to the informant's right to confidentiality occurs. Philosophers give three types of arguments justifying confidentiality:

A1 — A consequentialist argument is that if the information given in trust is not left secret the patient will not feel confident to divulge all private information that are relevant for the physician to arrive at a correct diagnosis. Hence, the best course of treatment cannot be provided to the patient.

A2 — This argument appeals to the respect for the autonomy and privacy of the person.

A3 — This argument is based on the doctor-patient relationship. By maintaining the trust of the patient when the patient has disclosed sensitive information, the physician is trying to live up to the expectation of the patient. If the medical oath includes a clause regarding confidentiality and the physician accepts it, then the patient has a right to expect fidelity from the physician.

None of these three arguments consider confidentiality as an absolute right. They are only prima facie rights and can be overridden under certain circumstances especially to protect a potential victim's life or to prevent significant loss to the patient or public.

Truth-Telling — Veracity or truth-telling is one virtue which has not been emphasized in the traditional medical ethics. Even the Declaration of Geneva did not mention the obligation of veractiy as part of ethical code of the medical professionals. It was in 1980 that American Medical Association very briefly recommended that physicians deal honestly with their patients and colleagues.

> Veracity in the health care setting refers to comprehensive, accurate, and objective transmission of information, as well as to the way the professional fosters the patient's or subject's understanding. — (*Principle of Biomedical Ethics* — Beauchamp and Childress, 2001, p. 284).

Respect for autonomy is the primary basis for veracity or truth-telling. We owe this respect to the person we are communicating with. All our communications are based upon an implicit promise of truth-telling. When a patient enters into a professional relationship with a physician, he enters into a two-way implicit contract. Just as the physician expects a free and frank disclosure from the patients, the patient expects an honest, accurate and objective assessment of his diagnosis, prognosis, risks, procedure of intervention, etc. The relationship between the doctor and the patient is based on trust, and truth is the basis of trust.

Problems of truth-telling usually occur when a bad news, such as a diagnosis of cancer or a prognosis of imminent death, needs to be given to the patient. There had been intense debate regarding whether such information should be withheld and if so under what circumstances. There have been shifts in the policy of disclosure. In a survey in 1998, 98% physicians were in favour of disclosure of the diagnosis of cancer to the patient compared to 88% in 1961.[2] The reasons cited were improved treatment of cancer, greater awareness, changed social attitude towards cancer and greater compliance of the patient.

Some physicians cited the wish of the family regarding disclosure. But if respect for autonomy is the basis of truth-telling, then this autonomy is violated by first informing the family about the diagnosis. A competent autonomous person may not want her family to undergo the pain and misery of her fateful disease.

However, truth-telling or veracity does not mean that disclosure should be made without taking into consideration other relevant factors. Age, emotional stability, current psychological state of the patient, etc. are important factors to be taken into account while making the disclosure. Sometimes only a partial disclosure can be justified on these grounds, and sometimes stage by stage disclosure is done to prevent harm to the patient. A sensitive mind, proper timing, a respectful approach and proper language are very important in making a disclosure to the patient so that the physician shows proper respect to the autonomy of the person while preventing any harm to the patient.

NON-MALEFICENCE

The Principle of non-maleficence has direct links with Hippocratic oath —

---

2. See Beauchamp & Childress, *"Principles of Biomedical Ethics"*.

> I will use treatment to help the sick according to my ability and judgement, but I will never use it to injure or wrong them. — (*Principle of Biomedical Ethics* — Beauchamp and Childress, 1994, p. 189).

It is a negative principle which imposes an obligation on the physician not to inflict harm to the patient intentionally either by act of omission or by act of commission. Its logical form can be expressed in the following way: "Do not do x," while the principle of beneficence requires the physician to perform actions that would not only prevent harm to the patient but also will promote her good.

Non-maleficence is a much more stringent principle than the principle of beneficence. It forbids the physician not to do any harm as well as not to expose the patient to any risks of harm.

In order to prevent harm to a patient a standardized system of care has been developed in the medical world. A case of negligence occurs when a physician fails to provide care to his patient according to this standardized care system. This standard requires proper training, skill, expertise and perseverance on the part of the care-provider.

Extremely important and controversial problems of withholding or withdrawing treatment come within the purview of the principle of non-maleficence. The problem of euthanasia, end-of-life care, doctor-assisted suicide, etc. are the controversial problems of medical ethics where this principle plays an important role.

BENEFICENCE

The dictionary meaning of "beneficence" includes acts of mercy, kindness, charity, etc. In context with medical ethics it enjoins the physician to actively engage in those procedures that will promote health and well-being of the patient.

This principle states that the physician should always act in the best interest of the patient. All emergency measures taken by the physicians are justified by this principle. In fact, many physicians believe that beneficence is the only justification for the entire medical system. The research, experiments, the treatment procedures and all the related paraphernalia can be justified only on the basis of benefit to the patient.

> " . . . beneficence provides the primary goal and rationale of medicine and health care, whereas respect for autonomy (along with non-maleficence and justice) sets moral limits on the professional's actions in pursuit of this goal. — (*Principle of Biomedical Ethics*— Beauchamp and Childress, 2001, p. 177).

Some physicians believe that as per the principle of beneficence, the primary duty of the physician is to act in the best interest of the patient, not to promote autonomous decision-making. Hence, if the decision of the patient conflicts with the decision of the physician, the physician is justified in ignoring it. This attitude is called paternalism.

> Paternalism is "Intentional overriding of one person's known preferences or actions by another person, where the person who overrides justifies the action by the goal of benefiting or avoiding harm to the person whose preferences or actions are overridden." — (*Principle of Biomedical Ethics* — Beauchamp and Childress, 2001, p. 178).

Paternalism refers to a governance by a father (In Greek, *Pater* = father). In medical parlance, paternalism is justified by pointing out that a physician has superior knowledge, skill, training and insight and this provides him with the authority to take care of his ignorant patient like a father does to his children.

Paternalism is of two kinds: strong and weak.

Weak paternalism shows some respect for the autonomy of the patient because it tries to protect the individual from her own harmful action that are substantially non-voluntary, such as a decision taken without getting adequate and relevant information, or a decision taken in a state of acute depression.

Strong paternalism tends to override the factor of autonomy altogether in order to protect the individual even though the decision might have been taken fully and voluntarily by a competent person.

Some philosophers have tried to bring about a compromise between the principle for respect of autonomy and the principle of beneficence by arguing that the best interests of the patient are often linked with their preferences. However, this may not be true in a large number of cases.

Supporters of paternalism also take recourse to a counterfactual argument. They argue that if the patients were rational, they would agree to the medical procedure decided by the expert.

There is a close relationship between the principle of non-maleficence and beneficence. The problem of euthanasia, for example, is a special ethical problem based on the principle of not doing harm to the patient. The solution of the problem depends on how the concept of harm is defined. If death is considered a harm to the patient, euthanasia cannot be justified on ground of the principle of non-maleficence.

Similarly, the principle of beneficence creates a moral obligation on the part of the physician to act in the best interest of the patient. The same problem of euthanasia can be viewed differently. It also depends on how the concept of "best interest" is defined. Maybe under certain circumstances withholding or withdrawing treatment is considered to be in the best interest of the patient. Thus, there is a large area of conceptual vagueness regarding the two principles and this often leads to controversy.

It is only recently that paternalism is being criticized. In traditional medical ethics or even fifty years back, paternalism was not considered ethically unsatisfactory. The general attitude was "The doctor knows best." However, the basic difficulty with paternalism is that it can justify any medical procedure without the consent of the patient on the ground that it was in the best interest of the patient.

JUSTICE

The principle of justice is an extremely complex topic and cannot be discussed in detail in this paper. The concepts of fairness, desert, entitlement, etc. are all attempts to explicate the concept of justice. Rawl's theory of justice and his concept of fairness plays an important role in modern medical ethics.

When we talk of justice, we usually refer to a twofold view: Individual justice and distributive justice. The former refers to the rights of an individual while the latter refers to a "fair, equitable distribution by justified norms that structure the terms of social co-operation."

In medical parlance justice require that if an individual has a right to receive health care benefits, it will be unjust or wrong to withhold it on the basis of caste, creed, religion or any other basis.

In these days of scarcity of medical resources, it is distributive justice that creates major ethical problems. How to distribute the scarce medical resources when the demand is greater than supply? If only one kidney is available for transplantation and there are three candidates to receive it, who should be given the priority? What principle is the "just principle" for making a decision? Should it be decided on the basis of age, or talent, or the social productivity of the recipient? Similar problems may arise in case of euthanasia. Is it justifiable to "waste" scarce medical resources for a comatose patient whose probability of survival is almost very low and deprive other patients who have high probability of survival with the help of those resources? Like all philosophical problems these problems are being hotly debated by physicians and philosophers.

In addition to these principles certain virtues and rights are considered important in medical ethics. I shall merely mention five of them:

i. Compassion

ii. Discernment

iii. Trustworthiness

iv. Integrity

v. Conscientiousness

As is clear these virtues would, to a large extent, determine how the patient would be treated by the physician. Apart from the principles, these personal virtues also determine to a great extent the quality of doctor-patient relationship and hence the quality of therapeutic interventions.

II

Let us now see how the principles stated above are affected by social and cultural factors. In India the code of medical ethics is not essentially different from the International Code. Since the Geneva Convention has accepted these basic principles, they are equally relevant in Indian scenario. In this section, I will discuss the ethical situation as it is currently prevalent in West Bengal.[3]

Informed Consent — In the current medical practice no informed consent is taken from the patient as delineated in the code of ethics in this paper. The patient or the patient-party (usually the relatives of the patient) is usually required to sign a declaration form in case of a surgery. If the patient is illiterate, their left-thumb-impression is taken on the form.

Patients are generally not directly informed of their diagnosis. Relatives of the patients are, however, informed of the diagnosis. Methods of alternative forms of treatment and the options open to the patient are usually not discussed. The course and plan of treatment is also rarely discussed.

Veracity or Truth-Telling — On my questioning whether they ever disclose bad news (such as diagnosis of cancer or prognosis of death) to the patient and if so how the disclosure is usually done, my informant responded that the physicians usually do not perform this task. The family of the patient is informed of the diagnosis and prognosis. The physicians leave the task of breaking the bad news to the patient on the family of the patient. This is especially true of a short survival expectation. The patient is usually never informed of the short expected survival by the physician.

When I pointed out that this practice consistently violates the principle of the respect for the autonomy of the patient,

---

3. I thank Dr. Deepananda Bhattacharya, Dr. Debashis Bhattacharya and Dr. Bhaskar Ukil for providing me with the information used in this paper.

they justified the practice by saying that it is not done with the intention of disrespecting the autonomy of the patient. The general educational level and level of understanding of the patients generally treated in government hospitals, especially in far-flung rural areas, is so poor that it is very difficult to explain to them the nature of the disease they are suffering from. It is also very difficult to explain to them the plan of treatment or the nature of therapeutic intervention. Also, they added, the mind-set of the kind of population they treat is largely of total dependence on the physician. The doctors are often treated like demi-gods and there is complete surrender to the plan of treatment decided by the doctor.

The doctors also justified their practice of not breaking the bad news to the patient. The bad news is usually not given to the patient in consideration of the psychological impact it might have on them. Thus, in this case beneficence overrides the principle of the respect for the autonomy of the patient.

As far as privacy is concerned total privacy is maintained regarding HIV-positive status of the patient. Even in blood-donation camps, if blood donated by a particular person is found to be HIV-positive, it is simply thrown away. Neither the donor nor their family/spouse is informed. It is the policy of the Government that the person should be shielded from the psychological trauma that will result from the knowledge of her being HIV-positive.

Confidentiality is, as a rule, thrown to the winds. Dr. Bhaskar Ukil sarcastically said, "Yes, we maintain so much confidentiality that even the patient does not know what is wrong with her."

The situation changes, however, with the kind of population being treated. Physicians are more careful in their treatment of the patient in areas where the educational level and the level of understanding of the patient is high. In private practice and in treatment offered in private clinics and hospitals, the situation seems a lot better. Dr. Ukil informed me that he routinely informs his patients of a cancer diagnosis. Sometimes he also informs his patients the extent of injury or damage to their system. He justified his decision on the following grounds: (i) it is easier to motivate the patient in co-operating with the treatment if they know what is expected of them in the process of treatment and why; (ii) a compassionate approach mobilizes the energy of the patient; and (iii) he does not consider it morally right to give wrong information to the patient.

However, in private practice also the bad diagnosis is often clearly discussed with the family of the patient, and rarely with the patient themselves. Since, in private clinics and hospitals the patient is paying a lot of money, they are entitled to ask questions. Even then the general attitude towards the physician is that of surrender and submission and the attitude of the doctors also is that of an authority. In those cases where the doctor is taking time to answer the questions of the patient and his family, it is generally due to the characteristic of the doctor's personality rather than as a matter of policy of respecting the autonomy of the patient.

If a patient, on rare occasions, requests a particular course of treatment not conducive to their benefit, the doctors would not accept it, informs Dr. Bhattacharya. Practice of euthanasia is illegal in India till date.

Compassion — Compassion is a rare "commodity" in government hospitals. The emotions of the patient are rarely taken into account while giving them bad news, such as, their child has Down's syndrome.

I did not have time to talk about the general practice regarding the problems of justice, but the main area of conflict is clear, that is, the conflict between the principle of respect for the autonomy of the patient and the principle of beneficence.

III

It is clear from the above account that the medical scenario in West Bengal (and probably in whole of India) is more tilted towards beneficence. Principle of respect for the autonomy of the patient has very little importance in the entire medical system. The Western medical system, particularly the American system, is largely guided by the principle of respect for autonomy. Not all Western medical systems, however, give priority to the autonomy or right of self-determination of the patient. While the liberal right-based approach of Western Europe gives patients the negative right to override the opinion of the doctor, the professional code of Southern Europe (called the Deontological Code) gives immense freedom to the physician to do what they think in the best interest of the patient. However, the doctors are enjoined to abide by the professional code of medical ethics. But once this requirement is satisfied, it is considered virtuous on the part of the patient to obey the dictates of the virtuous doctor.

Donna Dickenson writes:

> In Italy, for example, where codes of medical ethics date back to the Fascist period, there is a positive duty in the name of the collectivity to maximize one's own health and to allow the doctor free rein in the exercise of his or her beneficence. To the extent that this duty is positively enjoined on doctors, for example, by Article 28 of the Deontological Code, it would actually be morally wrong and legally

> dubious to stand in the doctors' way. Thus, if relatives of a handicapped person or child refuse consent to treatment, the doctor has a duty of beneficence to proceed regardless. Although the same article deals extensively with the patient's right to the informed consent, "in actual clinical practice doctors are given substantive discretion to resolve potential conflicts between the right of patients to be informed and the need to ensure their compliance."—Calzone, 1996. (*Three Different Models in European Medical Law and Ethics* — Donna Dickenson; *Cambridge Medical Ethics Workbook* — Michael Parker and Donna Dickenson, p. 286).

However, there has been a consistent shift from paternalism towards the right to self-determination of the patient. In the 1995 code, the old habit of informing the terminal diagnosis of a patient to his family but withholding the information from the patient themselves, has been done away with.

In Western Europe, the Netherlands comes closest to the American liberal model where the dominant emphasis is on the rights of the patients. Yet it is still significantly different from the American law.

There is no denying that all over the world medical ethics is giving greater importance to the patient's right to self-determination. As is evident from the above account the medical scenario of West Bengal, and probably in whole of India, does not seem very comfortable with the idea of the respect for the autonomy of the patient. Doctors do not like to be contradicted and want a free hand in following the course of action they think best in the interest of the patient.

I shall not go into the reasons why self-determination is becoming increasingly important in the current medical scenario. I shall very briefly argue that the principle of the respect for the autonomy of the patient is of fundamental importance in medical ethics. Principle of beneficence without the limitation set by the autonomy principle will give rise to undesirable forms of paternalism and morally unacceptable cases of medical negligence. However, my argument is not a consequentialist one. Following Kant, I believe that every human being has a dignity and he ought not to be treated merely as a means. Respect for the dignity of the patient alone can set limits to the paternalistic consequences of the principle of beneficence.

My arguments go like this:

1. Principle of beneficence enjoins the physicians to act in the best interest of the patient and to promote their good.
2. To act in the best interest of the patient is possible only when the patient is respected as a rational and moral agent, and not merely as means to some other end.
3. Without this respect for self-determination, the doctor can provide only clinical relief to the patient that may not be commensurate with the patient's view of what is in their best interest.
4. In such cases, even if the patient gets clinical relief, the doctor has promoted his own good rather than the good of the patient. He feels satisfied that he has performed his duties as per the principle of beneficence but he has not promoted the patient's good because some goods are related to the subject philosophy of life. Thus, the doctor has acted on the principle of beneficence but has failed to promote the good of the patient.

5. The principle of beneficence in order to be effectively implemented must be based on the principle of respect.

In most cases what the doctor thinks good for the patient is also endorsed or accepted by the patient. The patient generally accepts the superior knowledge and authority of the doctor. But in some complicated and serious cases this idea may differ and there is a conflict between the patient's and the physician's idea of what is good for the former. In such cases, acting only on the principle of beneficence might not be a moral choice. A decision based on a combination of autonomy and beneficence will be a more morally justified choice. This does not imply that in every such case the patient's idea has to be accepted by the doctor. The important thing is to treat the patient's opinion with respect — the respect an autonomous agent deserves. A solution of the conflict can be arrived at if there is proper respect on both sides. The autonomy principle does not imply that the doctor is bound to accept the opinion of the patient. Even autonomous countries sit for discussion on points of conflicts.

Take the case of Peter Knoll. He refused treatment because he did not want others to take charge of his life. He wanted to live a life where he would not be dependent on others — this was his idea of a dignified life. How can someone else decide what is in my best interest? A doctor is bound by his oath for the respect of life and would try to save the life of the patient as far as possible. But is saving life in all cases in the best interest of the patient? It is only in consultation with the patient, by giving him the relevant information, that the doctor and patient both can decide on a course of action. The doctor will provide the objective information, will recommend a plan, the patient will consult their own specific conditions according to their own philosophy of life. Therapeutic interventions based on such joint decisions alone can serve the best interest of the patient.

As I was writing this paper, there was a news flash on *India TV* (Breaking News, 26.7.2006, at 11 PM). A particular case of medical negligence was being reported by the media. Sayeed, an old man, came to one of the hospitals in Meerut for the treatment of his eyes. While waiting in the hospital, he fainted. The doctors declared him dead and he was ordered to be sent to the mortuary. The ward boy kept on telling them that Sayeed was alive but the doctors did not listen to him. While being taken to the mortuary, the ward boy noticed clearly that Sayeed was breathing. He called other doctors and pharmacists who declared him alive and ordered him out of the mortuary. The news anchor, Mr. Rajat Sharma, commented that this was the first time that a person who was alive was sent to mortuary due to the negligence of the doctor.

This, however, is just one incident of medical negligence. Cases of such negligence are galore in India. Cases of negligence and corruption in medical practice are the results of treating the patient as means and not as an end. If there is genuine respect for the patient, they will not be treated merely as means to some end, and cases of medical negligence will become scarce. There may be cases of genuine human mistake in diagnosis but cases of gross negligence are only the result of lack of respect for the patient.

Because of the frequent conflict between the principle of autonomy and the principle of beneficence, a number of alternative approaches are being developed in medical ethics. Also, dissatisfaction with the traditional theories of ethics, namely utilitarianism and Kantianism, has led to the emergence of feminist ethics, contextualism and particularism. Needless to say, the four principles of medical ethics are based on traditional theories of ethics. Rejection of these theories implies the rejection of principles in medical ethics too.

Virtue ethics, for example, views medical practice from the point of view of doctor-patient relationship. It emphasizes the importance of the character-traits that a doctor should possess in order to be responsible in that relationship, namely, honesty, compassion, integrity and justice. So, the doctor ought to tell the truth to the patient not because they have a right to self-determination but because the virtue of truthfulness is part of the doctor-patient relationship.

First of all, principlism does not rule out the importance of virtues in medical ethics, nor does it rule out the importance of relationship between doctor and patient as an important factor in the medical scenario. I contend, however, that respect for autonomy is more fundamental than virtues. The basis of virtues is a sense of respect for the person that forbids us to treat her with falsehood, with lack of compassion or in any unfair or unjust ways.

But will virtue ethics be able to solve the problem? As has been explained earlier, according to virtue ethics, the doctor tells the truth to the patient not because he wants to have her informed consent but because truth-telling is a virtue and he is a virtuous person. But then what would the doctor do in case of a conflict between compassion and veracity? If the doctor thinks that the patient will become disturbed on hearing a bad news and go in depression or have nervous breakdown, should he tell the patient the truth? If not, then he is acting on compassion and not on veracity. So, conflicts can occur in virtuous persons also and these conflicts are essentially of the same nature as the conflict between the four principles of medical ethics.

Social and cultural factors, such as the low-level of education of the general patient population, poverty, excessive work-load of the doctors, etc. that prevent the implementation of autonomy principle as discussed in section II, are contingent factors. These can be overcome with suitable modifications in the medical policy of the State or the country. Doctor-patient relationship based upon mutual respect is morally more acceptable than one based on paternalism.

3

Culture as Determinant of Patient-Physician Relationship in Āyurveda

Amit K. Sharma

THE notion of culture is so wide in its scope that it covers almost every dimension of human life. Ordinarily, the systems of beliefs, customs, conventions, and values which include in its sphere not only moral but aesthetic values also are taken collectively as a vague connotation of "culture." In this ordinary sense, cognitive endeavours such as science, mathematics, etc. and their direct consequences such as technology are put beyond the purview of culture. So from one point of view, culture is seen as those aforesaid human activities which are separated from the value-neutral activities of purely rational or cognitive search (rational here is used in purely cognitive sense). However, if we look at the cognitive enterprise closely we find an implicit value-system operating there which is neither different nor cut off from the rest of the value-oriented activities. Ordinarily, it is thought that science is culture-neutral and insulated from any kind of value consideration. This view does not seem to cover various aspects either of culture or of science. A deeper study of the growth of science discloses that the belief-system of a community and its values also play an important role in shaping his cognitive endeavours. Although some people think that there is no sense in talking about Indian science or western science since they are one, it is only a superficial position, and a close examination of the history of science compels us to read it essentially as a part of the history of that culture. The aim of this paper is to underline some of the important points of the development of science that are closely connected to man's cultural life. With special reference to Āyurveda an attempt has been made here to highlight this close link between culture and science that helps us understand how cultural factors determine or control scientific thinking.

The Relation Between a Vaidya and an Ātura

Ordinarily the relation between the patient and the physician is seen as a purely accidental and formal sort of relation. All human beings fall ill at one time or another in their life and for treatment they have to go to a doctor. It is obvious that the doctor to whom a patient goes for treatment may not necessarily be acquainted to the doctor earlier. From the doctor's side also it is not necessary at all. No doctor treats only his familiar patients. Any stranger may come to a doctor for the treatment of a sickness and the doctor has to treat him. So this relation is obviously an accidental and formal kind of relation but this cannot remain in this very form if the doctor sincerely wants to diagnose the disease of his patients and help him cure out of it. It is clear that merely the statements of the symptoms by the patient of his/her particular present problem cannot help the doctor to reach the cause of his/her disease. The doctor has to know about the patient's recent past and in twwhat connection he may have to also know about the patient's profession, family background, etc. A patient cannot disclose all these things before a person with whom he thinks he has only a formal relation. He has to have a little confidence in the doctor. This is a normal condition of relation between a doctor and a patient which is necessary for the treatment of disease. In Āyurveda (and in some other systems also), the relation between the patient and the doctor has to become a deeper one. The trust of the patient on the doctor which may only be a necessary condition for creating conducive situation for treatment has to deepen further as that helps the healing process directly. For a patient, a doctor is not merely an ordinary person who is merely professionally skilled but he is much more than that — he is next to God. The *vaidya* also has to look at the patient and treat him from a very different perspective. The *vaidya* does not look and examine the physical body of the patient only but he wants to understand the functioning of his life-force which covers the person's spiritual dimension also. Medicine and surgery, whatever may be necessary for the patient is done by the doctor to cure his disease by understanding all the dimensions of his existence, or the imbalance produced by various reasons. Examination of physical body is necessary and obvious but the examination of psychic and spiritual levels of a person's being is equally necessary for him.[1] So when a doctor examines a patient he looks at him not merely as a living organism but something deeper and higher than that. The patient also feels it clearly while the *vaidya* examines him. He knows by all the activities of the *vaidya* that he is trying to reach the innermost core of his being. This makes the *vaidya* in his vision somewhat an extraordinary person. He understands that his *vaidya* is very

1. *Śarirendriyasattvatamsamyogo dhārī jivitam* ॥41 ॥

   (A conjunction of body, sense-organs, mind and spirit is known as life). — ch.5, p. 1, *sūtrasthānam, Caraka Saṁhitā,* trans. vol. 1, trans. by *Āyurvedācārya* Sri Jayadeva, Vidyālaṁakareṇa Pranitya, Banaras: Motilal Banarasidass, 1947.

special who will give him the boon of restoration of *svāsthya* and he cannot repay his debt by merely paying him his fees. The relation between the patient and the *vaidya* is not merely a professional relation.

Significance of the Code of Conduct for the Vaidya

It is typically in Āyurveda that the *vaidya* is supposed to observe a code of conduct honestly. It is not necessary in any other system of medicine or therapeutics for the doctor to observe any moral code. As a normal citizen, everyone has to follow certain legal and social codes of conduct. The doctor, being one such citizen, has to follow them also but that code of conduct does not become obligatory for him because of his profession. In Āyurveda, however, a code of conduct is necessary for a doctor because of his professional position. He has to observe certain moral values strictly in his life. For instance, he should speak the truth, he should free himself from "I"-ness, he should not speak too much, he should not get either too happy or too irritated, etc.[2] Now, these values

---

2. *Na madyadyutavesyaprasangarucih̤ syāt, na guhyam vivranuyāt, na kancidajaniyāt, nāhmani syannadakṣo nādakṣino nasuyakah, . . . na catibruvata, na bandhvanuraktakr̥cardvitiyaguhyajñana bahiḥkuryāt . . . na dhiro na atyuccharitasasttvaḥ syāt, . . . navisrabdhasvajano, naikaḥ sukhī . . . na kāryakalamatipatyet, . . . neindriyavsagaḥ syāt, na krodhaharṣātanuviddhyat, na śokamanuvaset, na siddhavotsukyam gacchennāsiddho dainyam.*॥

   (Drinking, gambling and the company of prostitutes should be avoided. He should not make public the private secrets of someone. He should not humiliate anyone. He should free himself from "I"-ness, or personal ego. He should master the art in which he is trained. He should donate as much as possible. He should not oppose anyone. He should not speak too much. He should love all his near and dear ones and should never get alienated from them. He should not be impatient. He should not be →

have dual function in his life. Overtly, the observance of these values give him a respectable image in society and he becomes trustworthy for the people. Trust of a patient on his doctor is necessary not merely for his treatment. Trust also has a healing function for the patient. If a doctor is professionally very sound, that is, he possesses a good knowledge of human system and medicine but despite that if the patient does not have confidence in him then it is not difficult to envisage that it will adversely affect the process of the curing of the disease directly. Being trustworthy cannot be the substitute of the *vaidya*'s professional qualification but he has to have both of them essentially. Apart from his image of a trustworthy physician, the moral code of conduct enables the physician to achieve and stay at that undisturbed or non-perverted state of mind from where he could penetrate into the deeper levels of being and understand the cause of his ailment that surface at his physical or bodily level. Without such a mental state the *vaidya* cannot understand the complex psychic life or the subtle spiritual life of man.[3]

→ fluctuating or vacillating by nature. He should not practise anything which can hurt the trust of the people on him. He should always share his comforts and happiness with others; should be energetic and should never waste his time on unfruitful activities; should not get either too happy or too irritated. He should not feel too happy or proud on achieving success and at the same time should not turn gloomy at his failure. He should free himself from attachment, lust and greed.) — v.26,27,28; p. 72, *sūtrasthānam, Caraka Saṁhitā,* vol. I, trans. by *Āyurvedācārya* Śrī Jayadeva, Vidyālaṁakareṇa Pranitya: Banaras: Motilal Banarasidass, 1947.

3. *Kāryatattvaviśeṣagyaḥ pratipatto na muhyati* ।
amuddaḥ phalamāpnoti yadmohanimittajam ॥18 ॥

(One who is the knower of the true and real knowledge develops an attitude of indifference and non-attachment naturally. And →

Hence, the moral code of conduct prescribed for the physician in Āyurveda has also a higher epistemic value for him. It is not merely pragmatic.

The Behaviour of the Vaidya Towards a Terminally-ill Patient

It is important to note that in Āyurveda several indications are given to determine the death of a person. By a simple counting of rate of a pulse of a patient and through some other physical symptoms, the *vaidya* can ascertain whether a person is approaching death. He is even capable of forecasting the exact time of death. Apart from physical symptoms, some other indications are also given in Āyurveda that look like some sort of a superstition or a blind faith. Bad omens, whether they are superstitions or not is a separate matter. But it brings at least two significant points to our notice: (i) death is believed to be predictable in Āyurveda, especially about certain patients;[4] and (ii) death is not believed to be merely a cessation of the functioning of organism. Although it is the assumption of *jyoti-*

→ that detached person is a suitable candidate to eat the fruits of that true and real knowledge which comes as a result of detachment and indifference.) — ch. 18, p. 31, *vimānasthānam*, ibid.

4. *pramāṇamayusastvartheindriyamanobuddhiceṣṭādinanam vikṛtilakṣṇeirupalabhyateanimmitteih, ayamasmātkṣnanmuhurtaddivasatripaca* ।

saptadasdvādsaḥatpakṣanmasatsanmasatsamvatsaradva svabhāmaptsyate iti ॥

(If there appear certain peculiar and distorting symptoms in the sense-organs, objects of sense-organs, mind, intellect, and physical gestures, then it can be predicted that at what time the patient will die, that is, whether he will die the very same moment, the very next moment, after a day, after a week, a month, six months, or a year.) — v.165, *indriyasthānam*, ibid.

śāstra that the death of every man is fixed and predictable because his *āyu* (or living span) is fixed, in Āyurveda this belief is not comp2letely dismissed. Indirectly, in Āyurveda, it is accepted that death can occur because of various reasons; physical reason is not the only reason for death.

Whatever may be the reason for death, a *vaidya*, who is proficient in his skill, can know the time of death of his patient. Although he can know with certainty that his patient will not survive after his calculated period, he is not allowed to predict it before the patient. Āyurveda gives clear instructions to the *vaidya* never to inform the patient about his imminent death.[5] The reason for such an instruction is twofold. One obvious reason is that no ordinary person can remain healthy by accepting his death. All of us know, in general, that we will die but we never take it seriously till it becomes clear to us that it is imminent. This ignorance is a boon for a normal healthy life. The declaration of one's imminent death is so alarming for anyone that one cannot keep ones's mental balance after knowing about it. One might start sinking and might die before the predicted time of death. So a *vaidya* is instructed not to declare before his patient about his imminent death.

The second reason behind such an instruction is more important and significant. Āyurveda is a science which believes

---

5. *maranayeha rupāni pasyata api bhisagvida* ।
apṛṣṭen na vaktvyam pratupasthitam ॥61 ॥
pṛṣṭenāpi na vaktavyam tatra yatropaghātakam ।

(Even if he is sufficiently assured about the death of the patient, an able physician should never declare it before his patient without being asked. And even if asked, he should never declare it there where this news may become the cause of the death of the patient or be painful for the patient or his dear ones.) v. 61, p. 518, *indriyasthānam*, ibid.

in life and never loses hope for life. Despite his best calculations, the *vaidya* is not supposed to lose hope for the life of his patient. The spark of life may come from any source — may be an unknown mysterious source. By not declaring the death of a patient who is terminally ill, a *vaidya* does not foreclose the hope for his life from an unknown source and never allows him to sink before his actual death. It is to be noted that it is not merely modesty on the part of *vaidya* not to declare about the imminent death of the patient but it has a deeper reason behind it.

In other systems of medicine and therapy, a doctor is advised not to declare about the terminally-ill patient's death for a superficial reason only. It is the superficiality of this reason that nowadays doctors prefer to declare about the death of the patient because they think that it will help him prepare mentally for it. The attitude shows a rigid closeness about the system's own methodology beyond which no hope is entertained. Although a *vaidya* may perhaps more accurately predict about the terminally-ill patient's imminent death but he is not too close with his calculations to leave room for hope. He believes that despite his correct calculations, in some miraculous way, the patient can survive and live a longer life too. Āyurveda gives strict instructions to the *vaidya* not to declare the imminent death of a patient and to make room for hope.

The attitude of Āyurveda for life, death, and health is very different from other systems of medicine and therapy which depend heavily and centrally on observation, empirical tests and reasoning within the scope of such tests only. Life is not out-and-out material for Āyurveda; it essentially contains a spark of immortal divinity within it. Spirituality is believed to be the essence of every human being. According to the foundational philosophical belief of Āyurveda, any physical ailment is a result of imbalance between different *guṇās* of *prakṛtī* within an individual organism in the form of imbalance between *Tridoṣās*. Not merely physical and psychological, but there may be a spiritual cause also for this imbalance. Health and survival both are intricately related to this balance. Since spiritual reason is beyond the control of any *vaidya*, he cannot do anything about it. However, since he truly believes in the operation of this factor in human life, it is a part of his professional knowledge to enrich further his knowledge about it. Therefore, it is not merely modesty, or leaving some scope for chance survival but a sincere and integral belief of his knowledge that makes a *vaidya* look for some supra-earthly scope for the cure of disease also.

Although in *Caraka Saṁhitā* the *vaidya* is advised to have an indifferent attitude towards a patient who is terminally-ill, this should not be misunderstood as devoid of concern about his life and health.[6] An emotional involvement with such a patient may disturb the balance of the *vaidya*'s mind and it may prove to be an impediment in discharging his duties objectively. But it is important to note that the *vaidya* has an understanding of the life of the patient which does not finally end with his death. Death is merely a temporarily stoppage in the journey of the patient's life which extends beyond this life. In the back-drop of this understanding, the *vaidya* can take his patient's death with a calm and composed mind and also help the patient to develop such an attitude. In the absence

---

6. *maitrī karunyamarteṣu sakye pritirupekṣanam* ।
prakṛtistheṣu bhūteṣu vaidyavṛttiḥcaturaviddha ॥25 ॥

(Friendliness and compassion towards the sufferers, love and attachment towards the patient who can be cured and an attitude of indifference towards the terminally-ill patient — these are the obvious characteristics of a physician.) — ch. 10, p. 75, *sūtrasthānam*, ibid.

of this understanding, the *vaidya* cannot suggest to the patient to do that. If the doctor does not have any honest belief in the life after this life then he cannot preach the patient effectively not to care for his life without an apathy or cruelty towards him. Although in such a situation the role of *vaidya* changes to some extent, it is not opposite of what he was doing earlier. While giving all the treatment for the body, if the *vaidya,* whom the patient trusts, suggests to his terminally-ill patient not to worry about his ailment and prepares him to develop an indifferent attitude to his own body then it really helps the patient the way his medicines help him. The confidence of the patient in his *vaidya* produces that desirable effect which he cannot develop by hearing the same words from his near relatives or dear ones. It helps him withdrawing his attention from his physical pain; that actually brings down the level of intensity of pain. So, *Caraka*'s instructions to a *vaidya* to be indifferent towards his patient should not be confused with a pragmatic and professional attitude. It is full of compassion that arose as a result of his fundamental beliefs regarding his profession.

In fact, the patient-physician relationship in Āyurveda can be rightly understood only if we understand Āyurveda's fundamental assumption about human life and *svāsthya.* In this assumption, a proper importance is given to the spiritual life of the man, and his psychic and physical aspects of life are deemed to be integrally connected to it. Some elaboration of this point is necessary at this juncture.

The Spiritual Aspect of Human Life

The spiritual level of existence of human being is a necessary belief in Āyurveda. Man is not mere psycho-somata in the eyes of Āyurveda. Āyurveda is a system of medicine or therapy that has developed on a theoretical foundation directly based on *Sāṁkhya*'s philosophical assumption of *triguṇās*. Corresponding to three *guṇās* of *prakṛti* as explained in the *Sāṁkhya* Philosophy, Āyurveda assumes that the organism of human beings that includes his mind and intellect also are formed of three sorts of forces only. At every level of human existence these three forces operate. When they operate in a balanced manner then equilibrium is formed in different segments of the organism. But due to reasons, which may be both natural as well as supernatural, certain imbalances are created that result into diseases. *Asvastha* that literally means "not to be in oneself," occurs only when the balance among the three forces is disturbed due to any reason in any part of the organism. It is worth noting that this imbalance may be caused by some supra-natural factors also. All of us know that any living human being is not merely a combination of various natural components but essentially he is a centre of consciousness also, that is called *puruṣa* in *Sāṁkhya. Puruṣa* or consciouness is not a product of *prakṛti* — it is an explicit belief of *Sāṁkhya.* Unlike the materialist's philosophy, *Sāṁkhya* does not believe that consciousness is produced by nature or *prakṛti.* Consciousness exists in its purity having a full awareness of its identity. Its attachment to the objects of materiality or *prakṛti* produces *ahaṁkāra* that is its false identity and becomes the root cause of its bondage. The *puruṣa* — the individual centre of consciousness, has a spiritual aim within it. It has to liberate itself from *ahaṁkāra* and retain its real nature of a centre of pure consciousness. Within every individual consciousness, this aim is implicitly contained irrespective of his knowledge of it. An individual may or may not know that he has to regain his real nature of pure consciousness. In his life this inherent, implicit assumption manifests on various occasions in many forms. An elaboration of that point would prove to be a digression here. But, in brief, it would be necessary to point out that the general tendency of human beings of not being satisfied with his material achievements reflect his deep aspiration to achieve something beyond it which he himself does not know what? Through *svādhyāya* (or self-meditation) or by other means some individuals come to know clearly about his aim in life. A journey on this path forms the spiritual aspect of life. As it is stated that man is basically a centre of consciousness, it becomes clear that his spiritual aspect of life has a central importance for him. On this spiritual journey, the growth of the individual is marked explicitly and implicitly, in his physical and psychic life. This does not mean that a spiritual person's physical body grows in somewhat different manner; it is only to indicate that the physical body of a person does not remain completely untouched by his spiritual growth.

A spiritual factor of disease is a unique assumption of Āyurveda. A *vaidya* has to have the eye to see whether the disease with which the patient is suffering is produced due to physical reasons or spiritual reasons. If a person is on a spiritual journey and some disease is seen in his body because of the disturbance of the three forces in this process then the *vaidya* has to be cautious enough not to stop those symptoms to come up by the use of medicine which he would have used in the case of physical ailment. This situation arose in the life of Śrī Rāmakr̥ṣṇa Paramhaṅsa. Because of his spiritual growth, he used to feel peculiar pain in different parts of his body and despite all the treatments it could not be cured. Eventually, a *vaidya* who had this spiritual eye could understand the real reason of his disease and suggested that it should not be stopped from manifesting. He assured that it will disappear only when Śrī Rāmakr̥ṣṇa will achieve the spiritual height for which it was an intermediary phase of change. This actually happened in Śrī Rāmakṛṣṇa's life.[7]

---

7. Before the arrival of Bhairavī Brāhmaṇī at Dakṣineśwar, Śrī Rāmakṛṣṇa was suffering heavily due to a disease known as *gatradaha* in which his whole body burnt like fire. Mathurābābū took him to a number of *vaidyas* but it did not help. Śrī Rāmakṛṣṇa said, "from the rising of the sun till noon, the temperature of my body starts increasing and at 12:00 in the noon it becomes unbearable. I feel so uncomfortable that I enter into *Gaṅgājī* and stand there with water up to my neck for hours and cover my head and forehead with a wet cloth. Out of fear that I may end up in catching some other water-borne disease if standing there for hours, I come out of water, though unwillingly and lie down on a wet cloth on the marble floor."

   Brāhmaṇī thought otherwise about this disease of Śrī Rāmakṛṣṇa. She told Mathurābābū that it is not a disease. It is nothing but a by-product of the intense feeling of love of Śrī Rāmakṛṣṇa for God which has shaken him thoroughly at bodily level. Śrī Rādhā and Śrī Caitanya Prabhū also had undergone the same problem. There is no medicine to treat it. The simple method to treat it is to wear the garland of fragrant flowers and apply the sandalwood on your skin. Strangely, on the fourth day itself, this strange *gatradaha* was no more, p. 320-21, *vicitra kṣudhā and gatradaha;* ch. 22, *Śrī Rāmakṛṣṇalīlāmṛta,* vol. 1, Pandit Dwārakānath Tīwarī, Śrī Rāmakṛṣṇa Āshram, Nagpur. Furthermore, after a few days another physical problem started surfacing, but that also got cured with the simple method of Brāhmaṇī. Śrī Rāmakṛṣṇa said, "during those days I was feeling extremely hungry. No amount of food intake could satisfy my appetite. Whether it is day or night, I remained fully occupied with the thoughts of food. I started thinking from where now this new disease came. I told the whole story to Brāhmaṇī." Brāhmaṇī responded, "Baba, there is nothing to worry about. Those who move on the spiritual path to realize the God face this kind of problem at their physical level sometimes. Don't worry. Very soon you will be out of it." After uttering these words, she arranged various types of food items and sweet eatables in large quantity with the help of Mathurābābū and placed them in a room. "And then she asked me, "Baba, now you sit in this room and eat whatever you feel →

The spiritual or the supra-psychic aspects of human life plays a dominant role in giving him *svāsthya* at his physical and psychic levels. Āyurveda has pointed this out and shown a direction for research in this regard. A lot of research is needed to be done on this line. To understand *svāsthya,* in the backdrop of a spiritual philosophy, definitely shows how cultural life determines our thinking in this regard.

Conclusion

Indian society is seen as a caste-dominated society. The seeds of this caste system were present in the *varṇa* system of ancient India. Discrimination on caste line was, and is, a painful social reality of Indian society that cannot be denied. At times, the critics of Indian society take undue liberty to look down upon the Indian social system in this light. In such a caste-ridden society, the growth of knowledge is adversely affected. However, it is very strange to see that a science like Āyurveda grew on this land and was respected by all castes and classes of the society. It is a further surprising fact that grown in this sort of society, Āyurveda retains its pure objective scientific spirit by giving clear instructions that no discrimination should be made along the caste lines in the system. No one has been given a privileged position to study and practise Āyurveda on the basis of caste.[8] A student of Āyurveda has been

→ like to eat." I did the same and on the very third day that very strange appetite for food got cured." — p. 321-22, "Vicitra kṣudhā and gatradaha," ch. 22, Śrī *Rāmakr̥ṣṇalīlāmr̥ta,* vol. 1, Pandit Dwarkānāth Tīwarī, Śrī Rāmakr̥ṣṇa Āshram, Nagpur.

8. *Sudramapi kulaguṇasaṁpannam* ।
mantravarjamanupanitamadhyapyedityeke ॥5 ॥

(Even śudras who are prohibited to memorize the Vedic *mantras* and undertake *upanayana saṁsakāras*, are eligible to study and practise Āyurveda — this is the standpoint of honourable teachers of Āyurveda) — v. 5, *sūtrasthānam, Susrutasaṁhitā.*

instructed to learn his lessons from any competent *vaidya* irrespective of his caste.[9]

Gender discrimination also is seen as an old stigma of Indian society but Āyurveda does not make any such discrimination at all in this regard. Midwifery has been the oldest duty and privilege of women from the very beginning but the position of a physician was not generally granted to woman in any ancient system of medicine and therapy. In sharp contrast to this old male chauvinism, in India we find mentions of the name of many female *vaidyas* like Bhairavī Brāhmaṇī, etc. On the basis of above discussion, it would not be wrong to think that at least in a vital consideration of life and health, the culture of India was highly humane from the very beginning. Āyurveda did not make Indian culture. It was the Indian culture within which a rational scientific system of medicine and therapy like Āyurveda was evolved and developed. Had the cultural factors not been conducive and favourable for its growth, it would not have evolved. The age-old system of Āyurveda that is still successfully functioning and growing is a proof of the openness and humane nature of ancient Indian culture.

---

9. *Auṣadhirnamarupabhayama janate hayajapa vane* ।
avipaścaiva gopaśca ye cānye vanvasinaḥ ॥118 ॥

(Herdsmen, forest-dwellers, and other people who live in the proximity of nature are well aware of the medicines of their region by their name, form, and qualities.) — v. 118, ch. 1, p. 13, *sutrasthānam, Caraka Saṁhitā.*

4

Religion (Islam) and Sex
As Determinant of Physician-Patient Relationship

S.Y. Khan

Relationship — IT is defined as an agreement between two people who engage in some form of exchange with a view to accomplish certain goals.

Expectations

Patient — Needs to be heard, needs to express himself/herself, needs warmth and respect.

Doctor — Educated enough.

Models of Health and Illness	
Biomedical	*Biopsychosocial*
Dualist/Mechanistic/Reductionist/ Disease-oriented	Holistic.
Challenged by: Changing pattern of disease, and Escalating cost of health care.	

Before discussing the Islamic perspectives with regard to the psychological issues that arise in those stricken with critical illness, it is important to lay some groundwork regarding Islam. This is necessary due to the incredible ignorance that exists concerning a basic understanding of just what defines Islam in terms of doctrine.

Most of what will proceed about this topic will ring a familiarity to those who are acquainted with their own faith traditions — and this is by, dare I say, Divine design. This is true since Islam, in terms of fundamental beliefs and paradigms, does not claim to be a new or even separate "religion." Indeed, today's overzealous parochialization and rigid segmentation of things based on external appearance, including "religion," runs counter to the Islamic scriptural admonition to never allow "religion" to be a divisive issue. The term *religion* may safely be defined as that path that seeks a state of peace or submissiveness of the human self toward Divinity. This is what Islam exactly means in the Arabic language. One who practises this way is titled *Muslim.*

The term Islam and its lexical derivatives are used throughout the Qur'an. "Qur'an" literally means *recitation* — and is the title of what Muslims consider a revelation from Divinity itself in the Arabic language. This was a language spoken by the dwellers of the deserts of Arabia who were immeasurably attuned to the ways and realities of creation and the cosmos and developed an incredibly potent and rich language medium whose nuances and depth take years to master for even the greatest savants of language. It should be mentioned that Qur'anic Arabic is not at all the same as colloquial Arabic spoken today. The very sounds, cadences and words of the Qur'an are considered the Literal Word of God as either revealed directly, or through angelic medium, to a highly purified and saintly figure named Muhammad who lived in the seventh century in the Arabian Peninsula. One may often witness Muslim patients recifing litanies or passages of the Qur'an in an effort to unlock alleged healing powers that emanate from its authentic recitation. Anecdotally one may hear of positive results of such practices, and I am aware that studies have been done in an attempt to demonstrate their therapeutic value.

The Qur'an also defines itself as a scripture; in it we find the doctrine that Islam began with the Primordial Couple — Adam and Eve. The term *Muslim* is employed in reference to Noah and Abraham. Islam is considered that perennial way of peace and submission to The Sacred as practised by numerous saints and prophets mentioned in the Qur'an such as the above, as well as Lot, Isaac, Ishmael, Jacob, Joseph, David, Solomon, Job, Jonah, Moses, Aaron, John, The Virgin Mary and Jesus, as well as others. This way was crystallized during the mission of Muhammad, and those who follow his precedent have adopted the title Islam as a proper name signifying their respective faith tradition that encompasses ritual, law and spiritual development. The sentiments of Zarathustra of the Pārsi tradition, Buddha, as well as that which underlies the Hindu doctrines — all echo the sentiment of Islam as defined above. Hence the Islamic tradition embraces that which is authentic in all faith traditions; as an extension, the Muslim who understands her or his religion will theoretically feel at home with anyone who believes in One God, accountability of one's actions before Divinity and righteous conduct.

In fact, the Qur'an does not address itself to only those who follow the precepts of Muhammad, or Arabs, or the contemporaries of Muhammad; the call of the Qur'an is to any believer in God who wishes to deepen her or his relationship with The Creator. The Qur'an explicitly validates other faith traditions and recognizes that sincere practice in what is authentic in them provides legitimate vehicles to

Divine Proximity. There is no such concept as monopolizing Divine Grace based on outward labels or forms practised by any particular group or tradition. At the same time, however, Muslims consider that tradition which was elucidated by Muhammad as the most authentic.

From the Islamic perspective, there is no essential demarcation between sacred and mundane, or the secular and spiritual. All of life's activities are infused with a spiritual dimension — echoing as it were, Divine Remembrance — so as not to consider the material (including our earthly life) as an end unto itself. As testimony that this sentiment is characteristic of not only Islamic tradition, but also almost every traditional civilization, one often encounters the fact that healers have usually been well-versed in the spiritual dynamics of their respective faith traditions — many were even masters in these fields.

Certain themes arise in the context of serious illness that dive into the realm of religion. I will elaborate on some, namely — confrontation with self-mortality, coping with affliction and the desire for companionship.

Facing the prospect of one's own death and the subject of human mortality is a tricky subject. This is true now, more than ever, as today's pop culture exhibits a tremendously condemning aversion and distaste for mortality, which to a certain degree is at odds with most religious doctrine. Most faith traditions, including Islam, implicitly, explicitly and categorically highlight the relative transience of our earthly sojourn; they promote the fact that a greater reality awaits. This theme is recurrently addressed in the Qur'an. Many of the Prophet Muhammad's sayings (narratives and traditions known as *Hadith*) advise against deluding oneself into acting and feeling, as if this life is one of permanence. Among the sayings of various luminaries, one emphasizes upholding an attitude of a traveller who must traverse this life with care, always keeping the destination in view. These luminaries lived as such and they continually emphasized other-worldliness in their beings. An extension of that was to warn against succumbing to a *pathologic* attachment to the earthly phase of our existence. This attachment has many unfortunate manifestations — and often makes life difficult for us doctors.

Indeed, the very indices of real success and failure have little to do with what would be termed worldly and material indices of such, since material existence and progress are not ends unto themselves. Earthly life is to be enjoyed, but is important only so far as it *impacts* our spiritual development — either allowing it to soar to greater heights or degrade into misery despite an appearance of earthly success. Hence factors such as wealth, talent, fame, status, reputation, fortune, ego, pain, affliction, loss, hardship and misfortune can be seen as stimuli for spiritual evolution or devolution. The imagery of *trials* is often found in the Islamic tradition and ironically the saintly scholars are unanimous in stating that trial through misfortune is far easier to handle than *trial through fortune* — in terms of exhibiting the proper spiritual etiquette and growth before The Almighty.

In mentioning the term spiritual development we must examine the nature of human substance. The Qur'an alludes to the human being in several respects. There are references to our organic and embryologic composition, our physiologic and sensate faculties, our ability to speak, reason and contend and feel emotions. However, Islamic tradition goes further and adds to this, as the Qur'an clearly dictates that the quintessential defining characteristic of the human envelope is the soul (In Arabic: *Nafs*). This is a conscious, wilful, transcendental component of being, and the purpose of religion from an essential perspective is simply to guard, maintain and purify it. It must be emphasized here that there is no inherent conflict within Islamic doctrine between the physical, rational, emotional or spiritual components of the human being. Hence, there is no doctrine of harsh asceticism or turning away or shunning worldly aspects of one's identity, although there is recognition that the human condition is one of forgetfulness and distraction through worldly pursuits. It is also abundantly clear that most of the great spiritual masters in the Islamic tradition, including the Prophet Muhammad himself, chose a most austere, simple and non-lavish lifestyle — wholeheartedly content with a minimalist approach to material pursuits; moreover, during formal spiritual training under the guidance of sages and saints, there are times where restraint from worldly activities is called upon in an effort to re-harmonize the "components" of one's being.

For the Muslim and indeed any believer in most faith traditions, there is a sense of peace with regard to self-mortality. This thrust is often sensationalized, misused and misunderstood for a desire to seek death. Considering the maligning of Islam through contemporary geopolitical events and the tidal wave of woefully poor and infantile attempts at scholarship and journalism, I feel the need to explicitly state that on a concrete and doctrinal level, a Muslim does not seek death — but when it ultimately visits (as it always does), there is a sense of conciliation, rather than a horrid and even vulgar enmity. The Qur'an mentions those who look forward to meeting with their Lord. A famous traditional narrative recounts the death of a child from an undefined illness. The saintly mother informed her husband by asking what he thought of the fact that something precious they had been entrusted with was returned to its Owner. The implication here is clear. For the Muslim, life and its contingencies (such as volition and will) are a trust (Arabic: *amānat*) that is ultimately returned. Indeed, one of the Attributes of Divinity is *al-Hayy*, a Qur'anic term whose lexical field includes notions of "The Completely Alive" or "The Truly Existent" or "That which is Real Being" or "That which Fully Is." Our sense of being is but an infinitesimally pale reflection that subsists upon *al-Hayy*. Language buckles here, so I need to say that these words do not imply pantheism in any way, shape or form. Instead, it is an attempt to describe an utter state of dependence.

An aversion and discomfort with death may have multiple etiologies. From an Islamic standpoint some are valid. When the subject is a loved one, we encounter mourning a loss, closing a chapter of existence and missing an earthly presence. All are very real and charged emotional states that are respected. With regard to self, this sadness at the approach of one's earthly conclusion and want of more time to cherish that which is here and now, or fulfil responsibilities — these sentiments are embraced. But when the aversion and discomfort towards self-mortality and the general topic of death stems from an overattachment to material life and a delusion that worldly and material life is the end-all and be-all — this is criticized by Islamic doctrine. On a deeper level, the Qur'an mentions a certain type of aversion to death as analogous to a reflexive manifestation of a soul that fears a meeting with its Lord due to an intuitive understanding and witnessing of the negative qualities which have accrued on it via the damage it has consciously inflicted on itself.

To be on the lookout for a patient who wishes to open her or his door to remembrance is perhaps most critical.

So mortality is not necessarily an enemy. As a physician, I am very careful not to confuse mortality with morbidity, which is indeed the enemy. Morbidity and suffering are things to stamp out and alleviate and indeed can be thought of as separate from mortality. Many fear mortality because they confuse it with morbidity and suffering. Conceptually they are indeed separate, and uncoupling the two for discussion is mandatory in our context. There are many who experientially and quite firmly realize this crucial difference between mortality and morbidity — those in health care, those who are critically ill, those whose loved ones suffer through critical illness — these all understand that mortality can be an end to suffering. This again is a loaded topic, but the dichotomy between the two needs to be stated.

The next issue to address in dealing with this topic is the idea of coping — more specifically coping with critical illness. It is safe to assign critical illness under the rubric of trial and affliction in terms of formulating an understanding of a reaction to such states from an Islamic perspective. The first crucial premise to realize regarding our dealing with and reacting to conditions in terms of behaviour, formulating sentiments or action is that for the Muslim, the primary audience is Divinity. From a certain angle, the Qur'an is simply a recurrent medley on gaining an experiential realization of this notion. The Muslim is encouraged to always be in some form of *Zikr — a "remembrance"* of the vertical dimension to reality, even more — a remembrance of Divinity. One of the reasons for this is to surround oneself with *Zikr*. Directly extending from this is a care to maintain oneself in a state of proper *ādāb*, a term that includes meanings such as etiquette, posture, courtesy, approach, standing — all before the Primary Audience.

To summarize the Islamic perspective on coping, one can say that the Muslim is encouraged to struggle to alleviate affliction and hardship based on a sincere understanding of a given situation. The caveat is to maintain a sense of peace in one's inner no matter what the outcome of the endeavour is — success or failure. The very act of intention and effort, or in our case want for regaining health and coping with affliction, pain and therapeutics — these very things are indeed an end unto themselves, the results may go either way. This notion, among other things, is an acknowledgement of The Divine Will — which the Muslim knows is never capricious. Now what is it to maintain a "state of peace in one's inner no matter what the result?" Well, in the context of a successful outcome, it is to don an attitude or display the *ādāb* of *Shukr* — which essentially means *gratitude.* In the context of perceived failure of a struggle, it is to don an attitude or display the *ādāb* of *Sabr* — a highly charged term that includes meanings such as *patience, perseverance, fortitude, keeping one's chin up* and there is a hint of *resignation* in the term as well. There is a narrative tradition which states that the believers' heart ọn whatever level is perpetually in the *ādāb* of either *Shukr* or *Sabr,* and that life is a couple of days — one a good day (to express *Shukr*) and the other a bad day (for *Sabr*).

We need to explore the term *Sabr* a bit further since the struggle with critical illness obviously calls for it. It is indeed the hallmark for a Muslim when confronted with hardship. Implicit in the term is a struggle to ameliorate one's circumstances; hence, it should not be confused with passivity or fatalism. The term *Sabr* is used over one hundred times in the Qur'an. Recall that for a Muslim, the Qur'an is the Literal Word of God, and as a common saying goes, "God does not waste words." There are verses that proclaim that *God is with those in Sabr,* and *God loves those who practise Sabr.* Practising *Sabr* is seen as a most potent vehicle to Divine Proximity, for spiritual development and purification. There is an expression found in the Middle East: "May your hardship (or loss/trial/ affliction) be for you a source of nearness to God." From a converse angle, Divine Proximity is what the Muslim seeks; *Sabr* delivers such and necessitates the presence of hardship and affliction for actualization. Again, this is not to be taken to mean that a Muslim seeks hardship or affliction, but when the circumstances come around, there ensues a quest for *Sabr.*

The Qur'anic verses promising struggles throughout one's life are seen from this regard rather than a design by some whimsical and sadistic deity. Again we approach the impenetrable questions, as to the ultimate whys. The Muslim understands that to approach The Plan of God with the faculties of mental gymnastics is to approach taking in a landscape while blind, or to solve a multi-linear Boolean equation with simple arithmetic. However, there is a far more powerful faculty of realization and understanding for the Muslim, which when awoken renders protests of the mental and rational faculties into an annoying and irrelevant whining of a spoiled brat. The Qur'an refers to this as *knowledge or witnessing of the heart,* and it is this arena we are told the "why" is put to rest. This awakening comes only through Divine Proximity, and practising *Sabr* is a potential route. So, for the sincere believer, it is possible to come to terms with hardship and struggle, not so much through empirical deduction, reason, or discursive cognition, but through spiritual realization — at least this is what we are taught by the prophets and saints. For the secularist cynic, it is nothing but a self-serving fantasy and delusion.

Of course the ultimate inspiration for the practice of *Sabr* are the prophets and saints. For Muslims, the prophets (including Moses, Mary and Jesus) and the saints are pillars of *Sabr* and are forever an inspiration to those undergoing hardships. From the Islamic perspective, suffering from illness itself also contains within it a purifying and redemptive nature. There are traditions that allude to the pangs of illness being able to shed sins and spiritual pollutants as leaves are shed from a tree. This expationary Grace is operative with even minimal discomfort, such as injury that comes from the prick of a thorn. It is also functional in the suffering with chronic afflictions — epilepsy and blindness are mentioned, amongst others. The underlying premise to this pattern of thought is that it is far better to atone, purify, and rid oneself of spiritual pollutants here as opposed to dragging them with you in hereafter.

One absolutely crucial point to understand is that purification, spiritual development, atonement and expiation which comes in these scenarios and with *Sabr* is strictly conditional upon whether the subject allows Divinity into its consciousness. From the Islamic perspective, God does not impose upon the human consciousness; it is for the human will to accept or reject and hence there will be a rejection or acceptance of the Divine Grace. The following tradition illustrates this superbly: Prophet Muhammad visited an elderly Bedouin who had fallen ill and offered him words of comfort and prayed that his hardship serve as a source of blessings. The Bedouin didn't see it that way and scolded that his illness is nothing else than an entity whose pain crushes his very bones and whose fever boils his blood and hastens him toward a miserable death. Muhammad gently replied, "Then it is so."

From the Qur'anic standpoint, will and consciousness are not playthings in the least — the Qur'an makes mention of the fact that the heavens and the earth cowered from the proposition of being granted will and consciousness. Hence, from a certain angle, ones's consciousness carves out one's reality. Interestingly, the brilliant physicist and mathematician Von Neumann employed the phrase *consciousness created reality,* in acknowledgement of the way quantum theory and the new physics has overturned any attempt at explaining reality from an objective or truly empirical point of view. Yet how stubbornly and dogmatically many cling to their ideas of "the way things work" when it comes to ultimate realities and life's deepest issues.

Another element to keep in mind before we leave the subject of coping with illness is best summed up by the colloquialism, which states that sometimes things are "a blessing in disguise." This hardly needs any exposition, as almost all have been witnesses to this in their own lives — a time where hardship and difficult circumstances turned out in hindsight to be not such a malicious occurrence after all.

Since *Sabr* implies an intention and effort to ameliorate one's condition, it is little wonder that therapeutics are embraced. The civilizations that in the middle ages were spawned by Muhammad's influence (which in turn engendered many facets of this one) were noted for their advancement in the sciences and health care. Surgery, Medicine, and Pharmacology were established fields and industries. An Islamic tradition states, "For every ailment, there is a remedy — except old age." Hence strides in the fields of research and teaching were welcome. Cities like Baghdad, Cordoba, Damascus and Fez in the twelfth century had scores of hospitals dedicated to teaching, research, with wings for social work and medical students. More importantly, the lifestyle exemplified by the Muhammadan precedent (which was and is most often neglected) pointed to simplicity and moderation, emphasizing care in the diet (very pertinent these days considering the toxins that exist in industry foods) and meticulous hygiene, including oral. Muhammad was quite explicit in warning of the dangers of filling the stomach, as he stated that at its fullest, the stomach should be a third food, a third water, and a third empty. So from the Islamic perspective, preventative medical policies and evolving new therapies to combat illness is fully consistent with tradition.

Element to discuss in the context of critical illness is the desire for companionship. A sense of isolation is commonly felt by the afflicted, and visiting the stricken is a staple of Islamic social mores — and is indeed common to most traditions. One narrative relates that Muhammad had a neighbour who used to purposefully empty trash on Muhammad's doorstep and walkway. Once when Muhammad noted not having to wade his way through garbage — he was seen soon after at the neighbours' door enquiring about their health and asking if he may be of service — such is the premium of helping those who are ill.

At one level visitation provides comfort through sincere well wishing, sympathy, empathy, sharing, love and service. Most often, family is best able to actualize this and this truly is one of the blessings of familial love — so selfless and pure. Those who notice what happens to the elderly and chronically ill removed from family in extended care facilities experientially realize the importance of familial love and support and know there is simply no substitute for familial care. But visitation and companionship has a different level of meaning more geared for health care professionals and those in the ministerial fields. This has to do with what in the Islamic context is called *"Śohbā"* — a term denoting *companionship* and *presence.* When referring to *presence,* I speak not of the word in its secularized context, i.e. being in the same place in space and time. Rather *presence* as it is used in the phrase, "such and such has got a real *presence* about them." Authentic presence in the scenario of visiting the sick translates to an uplifting comfort, inspiration, love, encouragement, strength, exhortation to fortitude and even healing.

In the Islamic tradition, serving and visiting the sick is a vehicle for Divine Proximity for the visitor. There are numerous narratives that explain this.

We can conclude that for those who visit and minister to the ill with as much sincerity and *presence* as they can muster, there is a reciprocal dynamic exchange of Divine Grace and Mercy through which both parties are hopefully transformed. It is never a one-way street with care givers, be they an MD, RN, Nurse's aid, chaplain, or social worker. No matter how much they stumble, they tread the path of saints and prophets. However, if not possessed by proper attitudes, the situation may become downright disastrous, openly or otherwise. Despite appearances, it is an enormous task — hence the anguish, frustration and burn-out that exist side by side with epiphanies of joy and accomplishment.

5

Doctor-Patient Relationship
A Homoeopath's Appraisal

Swaraj Majumdar

IT doesn't matter if one believes in God or not, but certainly we have to have a philosophy of life — an ideal or outlook that ensures individual and collective growth which ultimately culminates in the realization of Truth or attaining fulfilment. The keynote of our Indian philosophy that rings through our various scriptures is this Absolute Truth. From the ancient Upaniṣads down to the later Purāṇas, including *Srimad Bhāgavatam* and The *Gītā,* all through you will find this exhortation — "Realize the Truth, realize the Truth." God is described there as *"satyasya satyam"* — "The Truth of all truths," *"Satyam param dhīmahi"* — "Let us meditate upon that Truth" — this has been the theme song of our spiritual literature. Therefore, if anything, we are the worshippers of Truth or Light. In the *Brihadāraṇyaka Upaniṣad* (II.1.20) therefore we hear this prayer: *"asato mā sadgamaya; tamaso mā jyotirgamaya"* — "From the unreal lead me to the Real; From darkness lead me to Light." But why don't we realize that glaring Truth? Because, says the *Kaṭha Upaniṣad, "Parānci khāni vyatrinat svayaṁbhū"* — "The Lord has made all our sense-organs outgoing." *"Tasmātparān paśyati nāntarātman"* — "Therefore, we are always mesmerized by the external, gross, material world and do not look within to find out the subtlest truth hidden there. Thus the finest, subtle, latent powers hidden in apparently inert objects elude us. When we find out that Truth we are fulfilled, for we have attained the highest. This Highest Truth has been described by our ancient seers, a *bhavaroga-vaidya* — the "Eternal Doctor" who can remove all our ailments or diseases called worldliness.

You may be wondering why I talk about philosophy, Truth, this and that! One may ask, "How are these at all related to homoeopathy? And how can these have any bearing on the issue, viz. doctor-patient relationship?" To answer all these questions we need to explain in a nutshell what homoeopathy is all about.

Homoeopathy — It is an art as well as a science. To put it simply, homeopathy, as opposed to many prevalent schools of treatment, is a wonderful art of healing. It may be likened to an *art* because it is not a painful and torturous device of beheading a patient in order to save him from migraine! On the contrary, it cures a patient without inflicting any additional injuries or pain on him/her. It just tries, and to a great extent, succeeds in taking off the suffering from the patient silently, gently and speedily without creating any adverse side-effect on his/her physical system so much so that often patients exclaim, "O, Doctor, that medicine you gave me the other day, had done a miracle! I took four sweet globules and my whole trouble disappeared!"

But, mind you, it's an injustice to call it a miracle. Why, miracle? It was bound to happen; it couldn't be otherwise because homoeopathy is not faith-healing, it is pure science as its results have been verified during past 200 years throughout the world and always verifiable by anybody willing to do so. The philosophy of this science discovered by the great German doctor Samuel Hahnemann is this: Man is not just a bundle of flesh and marrow, veins and bones. Behind his gross palpable physical body, there is a mind that is subtler than the first. But then, man is not a mere psycho-physical organism. There is still a third unseen dimension in him which is spirit. In homoeopathy, that invisible spirit is called *vital force.* It is not exactly Vedantic *ātman* or occidental soul, but I guess, it is a spark of it. When this vital force becomes deranged, we are overpowered by the disease-forces and suffer from various maladies. What homoeopathy does is to simply rouse and strengthen this vital force, chiefly with the help of minute doses of potentized medicines.[1] When the vital force or *prāṇa-śakti* becomes strong than the disease-force, the former routs the latter and the sick regains health. Here, a word of caution is also needed. This vital force shouldn't be confused with what is ordinarily known as the "immunity" system. This vital force is a far more deeper and comprehensive core of our being than the simple defence mechanism of our body which mainly consists of the anti-microbial action of the white blood cells and the formation of antibodies.

The doctrine on which homoeopathy is grounded unshakeably is *Similia Similibus Curentur* as enunciated by Dr. Hahnemann. It simply means, homoeopathy is the cure of "Likes by Likes." In other words, it is the "pathy" of "like sickness," because its medicines are used to cure only the exact conditions they can produce in the healthy sensitive individual. It instigates and records the effects of drugs on healthy humans who can provide the accurate information desired. Animals can't give us the symptom-picture we need. Such "proving" or test reveal their precise effects on human organs, tissues and *mentality*, before they are prescribed for the sick. Dr. Compton Burnett therefore styles homoeopathy as "The

---

1. In the *Gītā* (6/5), you find a *śloka*: *Uddharet ātmanātmānam anātmānam avasādayet* — "Raise yourself by yourself, don't let yourself down."

Scientific Medicine" because it is based on ascertained facts and abundantly proved deductions and not on any guesswork. A homoeopath's chief concern is to match the totality of the disease — symptoms with the totality of the drug-symptoms. That is why homoeopathy is commonly called a science of symptomatic treatment. If the symptoms of the disease and the drug correspond well, the cure is almost a certainty, of course when the disease is curable. When the disease has advanced too far and reached a terminal stage, for example in cancer, it will palliate and may prolong the life of a patient.

Nosology[2] or pathological names of diseases are not that much important in homoeopathy as it is in other systems because we feel no two cases are exactly alike and each case is a problem to be solved on the basis of symptoms. That is why homoeopathy can successfully combat a disease never seen before, but whose symptoms are known. This power of homoeopathy was displayed in 1830 and 1854 when cholera invaded Eürope and some other places. Only three medicines — Camphor, Cuprum and Viratrum Alb — valiantly saved hundreds of lives whereas other systems, whose approach was entirely clinical, failed miserably.[3] Only a few years ago the world was shaking with fear of anthrax poisoning and early last year people of West Bengal got terrified by the sudden onset of dengue, many even lost their lives. Thanks to homoeopathy, our drug-arsenal is potent enough to combat any such crises. We don't have to wait in such circumstances for the detection of the mysterious "virus" or some such thing.

---

2. A clinical approach is also there in homoeopathy, but it is a secondary approach, although its value can't be absolutely disowned. Dr. John H. Clarke and others of Britain have stressed this point.
3. For details, see *British Journal of Homoeopathy*, 1854, pp. 521, 686.

We can safely and confidently prescribe the appropriate medicine on the basis of the totality of the patient's symptoms and cure the sick.

Homoeopathy's approach is holistic. Therefore, in a sense, it doesn't treat the disease, it treats the patient as a whole. It takes into account not only the patient's physiological symptoms, but also his/her mental symptoms, if not also spiritual symptoms. Science discovered long ago that man is a body-mind complex. But thousands of years before that, Indian *ṛṣis*, without the help of sophisticated instruments, realized and declared that man is not only a body-mind complex, his nature is essentially Spiritual or Divine. So, in the treatment, all these three layers of human personality have to be taken into account. Hence, homoeopathy attaches more importance to patient's mental state and his/her mental symptoms which more often than not provide wonderful clues to the roots of the disease and its single panacea. For example, if someone suffers from a fixed idea as if a strange person were at his side, or a living animal were in his abdomen, this queer feeling will point to a medicine called Thuja Occidentalis. Or again, if a patient is indescribably despondent and talks of committing suicide, the drug-picture of Aurum Metallicum will flash immediately into the homoeopath's mind. These curious sensations and bizarre feelings are ordinarily overlooked or rejected by other systems of medicine as being of no consequence. They are considered mental constructs of the patient. They are ruled out as baseless imaginary feelings. But to a homoeopath, these subjective symptoms are pure gold. These are also very much real to the patient. We don't claim we know why they feel that way, but all the same we know what to do and how to help the patient to overcome that disturbing and troublesome "mania." This is one of the many plus-points of homoeopathy. It is interesting that even some allopaths have started realizing this point. Dr William Pullen, Clinical Assistant Professor of Medicine at the University of California, has recently stated that "Treating the body without acknowledging the mind and soul fails to take proper advantage and often threatens harm."[4]

Another thing in this connection must be mentioned. homoeopathic approach being holistic, a homoeopath collects all the symptoms that cover the entire body of the patient in a definite anatomical order, technically known as the Hahnemannian *Schema.* While he gives special attention to the primary ailment which is most distressing to the patient, he keeps his eyes quite open to the secondary disorders also, if there are any. For example, a patient comes and tells the doctor that she has been suffering from a pain from sacrum to the pubis and her M.C. (menstrual cycle) has stopped two months ago as she has conceived. The physician is also told that she can't just stand any music which made her intensely nervous. What the doctor does in this case? May be he will give a medicine called Savine that stops the pain as well as makes music tolerable to her. The patient is thus spared from going to a gynaecologist and then to a psychiatrist. So, it is economic in every sense, especially in a country like India. No other system, I believe, can offer such comprehensive all-round treatment under one umbrella.

Patient-Doctor Relationship

Against this backdrop, let us now examine the various facets of patient-doctor relationship. First we will discuss the relationship prevailing generally in the medical field

4. "Reflections on suffering," *The Key to a Meaningful Life,* Sri Ramakrishna Math, Uad . . . 1996, p. 182.

irrespective of "pathics" — homoeopathy or allopathy[5] — and then we will see what kind of problems a homoeopathic physician and his/her patients face and how the distinctiveness of homoeopathy influences that relationship in particular. But before we proceed let us acknowledge the fundamental fact that the relationship between a doctor and a patient depends largely on the doctor's ability to cure the disease of the patient. As this ability varies from doctor to doctor, from case to case, so is the relationship coloured and regulated by the support and amount of relief each patient gets from his/her doctor in moments of suffering. The maxim that "Nothing succeeds like success" is the rule of the game here. When a doctor cures an apparently incurable patient and brings him/her back from the jaws of death, as it were, the doctor appears in the patient's eyes as God in human form — *Vaidya Nārayano Hariḥ.*

This applies to homoeopaths, allopaths, āyurvedic *vaidya*s or physicians of any school. Thus, besides money, the physician also is rewarded with the patient's trust, confidence and appreciation. The physician's own job-satisfaction, of course, is the greatest here. An ancient Sanskrit verse therefore says, *cikitsā nāsti niśphala.* "A physician gets," says the verse, "sometimes *puṇya,* sometimes friendships, sometimes money, somewhere else fame and often knowledge and experience. Never is treatment without its fruit."

Śrī Rāmakṛṣṇa classifies physicians into three groups — *adham* (inferior), *madhyam* (mediocre) and *uttam* (superior), and reveals their respective concern for and relationship with their patients. He says:

---

5. The term "allopathy" means curing of a diseased action by inducing another action of a different kind. Homoeopathy is exactly its opposite.

> "There are three classes of physicians: superior, mediocre, and inferior. The inferior physician feels the patient's pulse, merely asks him to take medicine, and then goes away. He doesn't bother to find out whether the patient has followed his directions. The mediocre physician gently tries to persuade the patient to take the medicine. He says: "Look here. How can you get well without medicine? Take the medicine, my dear. I am preparing it with my own hands." But the superior physician follows a different method. If he finds the patient stubbornly refusing to swallow the medicine, he presses the patient's chest with his knee and forces the medicine down his throat."[6]

What Śrī Rāmakṛṣṇa in his characteristic witty manner remarked more than 125 years ago regarding different attitudes of doctors, still hold true, though the days of family physicians out on their visits to patients' houses have become a thing of the past. Personally I feel, in certain respects, those were the golden days when the doctor knew almost each and every member of the family by name and their constitutions. So, whenever he would go to see a particular patient, he enquired about the other members' health and give necessary advice if their health so demanded. In this way, a warm social relationship grew between doctors and members of the patient's family. Both from medical and social point of view that was a very healthy feature. I personally remember an allopath with great reverence and love. He was our house physician and happened to be my friend, philosopher and guide in my youth. Apart from his professional skill, his personality was inspiring; he cared for the poor and the sick; he would visit any patient in the neighbourhood even when

---

6. *The Gospel of Śrī Rāmakṛṣṇa,* Red-letter Edition, 2000, Sri Ramakrishna Math, Chennai. pp. 865-66.

he was called at dead of night. That dedication, that spirit of sacrifice is rarely seen nowadays.

One may argue that the number of patients has increased so much that doctors have little time to cultivate such sweet and human social relationships. But that is no answer, because the number of doctors has also increased proportionally, especially in urban areas. Very rarely doctors are willing to respond to a house-call, not to speak of a nocturnal visit! They generally tend to advise that the patient should either be brought to his clinic or, if the condition is serious, he should be hospitalized immediately. But where are "hospitals" nowadays? A few old such institutions are still there, but they are languishing for hundreds of reasons. Then, what to do? Send the patient to scores of well-decorated and well-designed private clinics and nursing homes scattered here and there in the metropolis (In the rural areas, conditions are more horrible, because such clinics are rarely seen in remote villages!) which are without senior doctors except at fixed hours of the day. In many cases you have to depend on junior doctors, or you have to contact a senior doctor, of your choice from outside and request him to carry on the treatment. Such is the general situation today! What kind of relationship will grow in such a dismal atmosphere except bitterness and frustration?

Then, these are the days of specialization and specialists! None can deny their importance. We need them very much, but only when *we really need* them. In chronic cases of serious nature or in seriously complicated acute cases where life is under great risk, we have to consult them and seek their expert service. But in acute cases of ordinary nature we hardly need them. Of course, one is absolutely free to consult a specialist for each and every problem if he has the means and will to do so. But that is individual choice and not a compulsion.

However, an impression is being artificially and purposefully embossed on the psyche of a patient by interested quarters and media that for every complaint they should rush to a specialist or their life may be in danger. Therefore, if one suffers simultaneously from acne, anaemia, insomnia and tonsillitis, one has to go to a dermatologist, hematologist, neurologist and to an otolaryngologist in succession. In the absence of a comprehensive treatment, the patient swings ceaselessly from the court of one specialist to the other. How an abiding doctor-patient relationship can thrive in such an uncertain and fluid situation? Neither the average doctor seems to care for the patient except suggesting a number of routine tests and dishing out a prescription within the shortest possible time, nor does the patient care for the doctor when the treatment is over. If you are cured, you don't come back to the doctor and offer your thanks. And if you don't get any positive result, you possibly curse him from a distance and rush to another specialist! There are always a few exceptions, but that is generally the pattern of doctor-patient relationship today.

As I have pointed out in the first part of this paper, homoeopathy is a system of medicine in which comprehensive treatment is possible. The same doctor will take care of your number of problems at a time. And since homoeopathy is symptomatic treatment, the doctor allows a patient to tell his/her own story of suffering uninterruptedly. He is never discouraged to express himself, on the contrary he is encouraged to do so. A good and conscientious homoeopath must be a good listener who should give at least half an hour to each patient, or he will fail to gather all the symptoms and formulate the diseased's correct picture. I knew a homoeopath who had a roaring practice, and he was my teacher, who didn't give more than two minutes to a patient! I told him once, "Sir, this is not homoeopathy, this is something else!" Anyway barring such instances, homoeopathy usually offers both doctor and the patient greater scope to know each other well. The doctor knows the patient from head to foot including his temperament and the history of his past diseases. So gradually a relationship based on mutual trust and confidence is likely to develop.

This, however, is not to suggest that there are no inhibiting factors. There are. Yes, in homoeopathy too. For example, some patients who love to guard their privacy, are often disturbed when the physician asks him too many close questions like Sherlock Holmes. Such patients are usually newcomers and they have had no previous experience of being treated homoeopathically. So they raise eyebrows which seem to say: "Non-homoeopathic doctors never asked me such questions! In a minute or two they heard my complaints and handed over a prescription. Why are you so inquisitive about my personal life?" If you can't convince such patients, they may never turn up to you in future. But you have to take it and stick to your principle.

Then there are patients who dislike the fact that the doctor gives them too small dose of a medicine. "I took four or five kinds of tablets daily for years; yet my trouble persists. And you say, four globules twice a day, will cure me in a week?" If the patient tries the medicine, he will in all probability come back to the doctor for his future ailments. But if he doesn't trust the doctor, he will never try the medicine and never return! He will get into his old groove!

There are also other minor impediments such as self-medication and surface-knowledge of homoeopathy. Self-medication, if not continued for too long, may not be harmful, but it is bound to be ineffective if disease-symptoms do not match drug-symptoms. Very often old patients recommend such medicines to others expecting that the medicine that helped them very much in the past will also help their friends and relatives. When that doesn't happen, the latter calls homoeopathy into question and the physician, who originally prescribed the drug to his patient long ago, is put to disrepute. Similarly, surface-knowledge of homoeopathy may also create misunderstanding with the physician. For instance, if such a patient is given "Tuberculinum" and he has read some elementary book on homoeopathy, he may feel insulted and ask in exasperation: "Doctor, do you think, I'm suffering from tuberculosis? It is impossible!" Having said this, he may leave your chamber in a huff, never to turn up again, and may think "homoeopathy is all bash!"

Conclusion

In conclusion, I want to stress the fact that man has grown so individualistic and self-centred today that no relationship is durable. I am for you so long as you are for me! Family bonds are breaking very fast. Marriage has become a matter of convention and convenience and not an emotional necessity and commitment to elevate oneself to higher planes of life. Faith in all ideals and ethical values are eroding in this materialistic, consumerist "civilization." The predominant urge is for one's self-gratification and to posses more and more, and this inhuman tendency is relentlessly fuelled by the media and business organizations throughout the world in their own interests. In this unstable socio-political and economic milieu, how can the doctor-patient relationship run on an idealistic course? Dr. B. Ramanath, a leading neurosurgeon, has recently regretted in an article that "there has grown an increasing tendency amongst doctors to adopt measures that are not always for the good of the patient. This has produced in the public mind a mistrust of the medical profession." But then, he goes on to say that "to expect the medical profession alone to be pure milk in an ocean of salt water, is unrealistic."[7]

The remark is only very true. Unless the ethical attitude of the society as a whole doesn't improve, the patient-doctor relationship is bound to suffer like every other relationship. It is a vicious circle. But how to break it? With the help of Consumer Protection Act? The Act has its necessity and utility, no doubt, but it also has increased psychological stress on physicians and the cost of treatment has escalated to dizzy heights. Then, what is the way out? Health Maintenance Organization (HMO) — a pre-paid Managed Care, as doctors like R.D. Lele suggest? Dr. Lele suggests that HMO providing a pre-paid managed care linked to health insurance, is the new paradigm for health care in the 21st century. According to him, the medical community assumes leadership and accepts responsibility and accountability in the HMO concept.[8]

I think the true solution lies in upholding our perennial Indian ethics that is embedded in Vedānta philosophy, a philosophy which emphatically declares that man is essentially Divine, and not a mere "consumer." To bring down Divinity or even humanity to the level of a consumer! What a horrible degradation we have brought ourselves to! Not simply money-earning or merely professionalism should be the motive of a physician. The motive should be service or *seva.* He should bear in mind that his nature is Divine and his patient is also divine in essence. Therefore, he is one with his patient. In other worlds, he is serving himself, and it is a great privilege

---

7. "Values in the Medical Field," *The Key to a Meaningful Life*, p. 172.
8. *"Advanced Health Care for All,"* by R.D. Lele, The Ramakrishna Mission Institute of Culture, Kolkata, 2005, pp. 12-13.

to do so. Physicianship is not just a money-earning and status-winning profession, it is one of the noblest missions through which one can manifest Divinity, his ultimate goal. It is a mission through which God gives His healing touch on the sick and the suffering humanity. Let us not forget that Swāmi Vīvekānanda, the greatest modern Vedāntist, therefore said: "Let the giver kneel down in all humility and thank; let the receiver stand up and permit"[9] If we, physicians of all denominations, can catch only a spark of this Vedāntic spirit, the entire doctor-patient relationship will be revolutionized.

Let us be humble, let us be patient and modest. Let us not emulate others' weaknesses. Let us try to be as perfect as possible and set examples which others might follow.

---

9. Swami Vivekananda, *Complete Works,* Mayavati Memorial Edn., vol. 7, p. 68, Advaita Ashrama.

6

Concept of Indigenous Medicine

Sashinungla

THE study of traditional medicine includes articulating an indigenous knowledge approach to understanding what traditional medicine is and why it historically existed outside dominant institutions, biomedical models and Eurocentric paradigms. The Report on the Protection of Heritage of Indigenous People defined, "Indigenous knowledge as a complete knowledge system with its own epistemology, philosophy and scientific and logical validity . . . which can only be understood by means of pedagogy traditionally employed by the people themselves." — (Battiste and Henderson, 2000).

Indigenous knowledge structures are like scientific theories in that they generalize from concrete experience, but unlike theories they are not systematic formulations of laws or methods. Rather, they involve the adjustment of forms of human livelihood to the environment in which they are embedded (Atran, 1999). The idea that indigenous knowledge must be science, because it leads to empirical results consistent with western science, is based on a concept of nature as a "pre-given" and "science" as the only means of discovering its universal laws (Berlin, 1994). Pushing indigenous knowledge into the framework of "science" is to discount an objective reality independent of human experience. People formulate their worlds by their knowledge and live by it. Therefore a philosophy of knowledge should implore how these varieties are variously produced, represented, transmitted and applied.

The indigenous medical practice has sustained in society's socio-cultural complexes through deeply rooted processes. It is a set of concepts of health, sickness and healer-patient relationship that reflect certain values, traditions and beliefs based on people's ways of life. The term "traditional medicine," as identified by the World Health Organization:

> is the sum total of knowledge, skills and practices based on the theories, beliefs and experiences indigenous to different cultures, whether explicable or not, used in the maintenance of health as well as in the prevention, diagnosis, and improvement of treatment of physical and mental illness.[1]

The physician-patient relationship and interaction is a central process in the practice of any medical tradition. There are many perspectives from which to understand and describe it. In different societies, periods and cultures, different values may be assigned different priorities.

The indigenous medical practice of the Aos of Nagaland like other ancient healing systems in the world is firmly based on personalistic tradition of supernatural "healers,"[2] *nemtsur* (bonesetter/herbalist), *rajenlar* (diagnoser), *tia-sār* (ritualist-

1. World Health Organization, Report 2001.
2. A common term used by anthropologist is "shaman" to cover herbalists, traditional healers, diviner and priests of native people. Originally, it referred to the way Tungus (a Siberian people with linguistic ties to the Manchurians) referred to those individuals responsible for the health of the community and their relationship to the supernatural world.

diviner/spiritist) and *temhi-lier* (tigerman). Thus, indigenous Ao medicine is an umbrella term that encompasses the healing beliefs and practices of their people. It is a holistic healing approach that emphasizes the treatment of body, mind and spirit. Aos believe that the health of an individual is inextricably linked to the people and objects surrounding that person, and that illness emanates from a disjunction of quasi-equilibrium maintained between man, his environment and the supernatural. Therefore, their healing practices is aimed to promote harmony among everyone in a community — and with the physical environment and the spiritual world as a whole.

In other words, Aos believe that all things in nature are interrelated (Sashinungla, 2005). They also believe that every human and every object has a reciprocal presence in the spirit world and that spirits can promote health or cause illness. Therefore, spiritual rejuvenation and the achievement of a general sense of physical, emotional and communal harmony are at the heart of indigenous Ao medicine. This restoration of the balance or the return to health can only be attained through a "healer."[3]

Since a person according to the Aos is simultaneously a body, a self (psyche) and a social being, a *rachenlar*[4] attempts to resolve the sickness caused by the disorder of the "social self," and also claims to cure diseases which arise from disorders of body by means of an elaborate diagnostic system. Social or cultural-bound syndromes referred as *kitsung* or

---

3. A healer whose power may be inherited from ancestors, transmitted from another healer, or developed through initiation.
4. In this paper word *rajenlar* is being used in a general sense to cover the terms shaman, healer, medicine man, etc.

"deity's illness"[5] are generally treated by *amempong* or ritual cleansing ceremonies, and physical ailments by *nemtsuba* or through administration of herbal extracts.

The specific healing procedures utilized in Ao indigenous healing slightly differ from one village to another and from healer to healer. However, the varying causes of disease are always considered, including the persons' past deeds, their state of mind and emotions, and whether they are in or out of harmony with the spirit world.

Accessibility of different healers enables them to switch from one type of healer to another in search of the best. Thus, they employ pluralistic strategies not perceiving any conflict among these alternatives, nor do they seem to perceive them as different systems, but rather as a variety of options, among which they can choose. Though very popular, they lack 'official' status as in many other tribal medical tradition all over the world. They operate within the socio-religious paradigm. It is simulated that these are sanctioned by their socio-religious beliefs. Thus, it works on the individual healer's methods, reputation and performance. In other words, the traditional healer's role stands at the interstices of religion, spiritism and social system and gains its power from this position.

These spiritualists and diagnosticians also intervene on the community's behalf and prevent disaster or calamities — a practice that often involves communication with the spirits, the supernatural and the physical entities that assist in the diagnosis. They are often the "seers" or communicators through ceremony who identify the ailments, remedies or ceremonies that are required to restore good spiritual,

---

5. Illness such as bodily pains, indigestion, headache, etc. are attributed to the annoyed spirits.

emotional and physical health, and well-being of the whole community.

As far as the relationship between the healers and the patients is concerned, there is no distrust and traditional healers are highly respected for their powers and service. They are not only highly revered for their expansive knowledge of cultural and spiritual practices but also for their devotion, commitment, sanctity and consecration. Their primary focus is on the well-being of the people. Thus it is normative for these individuals to sacrifice their daily lives to rituals, prayers and healing. Such is the trust and belief the people bestow on them that even if the patient dies in spite of the *rachenlar*'s efforts, the blame is passed on only to the evil spirits, but never to the *rachenlar*.

In spite of all these powerful and supernatural influences from *rachenlar* in the Ao cultural and community life, the ordinary people, even after seeking their help, never bowed before them in any gesture of worship (Imchen, 1993). Neither do the *rachenlar* claim nor demand any adoration or special status from the people they live their life with like any ordinary people. Even they do not charge anything in terms of material or money from the patients for their service.

It is imperative to make clear that in Ao society, medical knowledge never existed as an autonomous and formal body of knowledge. So also the healer-patient relationship is not founded on any fomulated criteria or guidelines. It is more of a "shared world-view" based on trust and belief. Or if there exist any such criteria or guidelines expected of the healer-patient for the success of the treatment, then it is the faith, trust and loyalty of the patient towards the particular "healing" that is being undertaken. Again, it is interesting to note that trust, faith and loyalty here is indicated towards the very practice but not necessarily on the healer. This is a tricky one, as the Ao healers are believed to be endowed with some supernatural sense. Excerpt from an interview:

> Healer (a Tigerman): Oh no! How can you be healed if you have no faith? (feeling the palm/forehead of the patient by his hand). You had gone to them (referring to modern physician) and now it is all complicated . . .[6]

Another significant role of an Ao *rachenlar* is that he fulfils the duty of "warding off the attack of evil spirits." Normally, a *rachenlar* is called in by the patient's family to diagnose the nature of the sickness by a "unique process" before he attempts to cure it. However, it is never the case that a healer will attempt to direct his supernatural powers against any patient, community or situation. In fact, to be gifted with such powers is considered by many *rachenlars* as a very demanding "responsibility given to them" that involves sacrifice and self-denial for the service of the people. One of the reasons cited by the healers is that while attending to a patient it is expected of them to "abstain themselves from the worldly things" and must "keep holy and pure" in order to make the diagnosis and rituals "acceptable" to the spirit.

The holistic approach of the Ao medical tradition is both its brilliance and its ultimate complexity. The natural environment shapes the medical expertise and practices applied by them. It is highly localized and it is social. Their epistemology is tied to the land, the spiritual laws that govern that land, and how co-existence between animal, plant and

6. Reproduced here is an excerpt from the series of interviews the author had with those healers of the Ao area of Nagaland to substantiate the point.

human life interrelate to a collective balance. Their "ethnoscience"[7] reflects the uniqueness of the place and, thus, their knowledge of traditional medicine is intrinsically tied to the land and revealed through language and culture.

The healer is central to the process of symbolic healing, and in this sense the Ao healers are central to their indigenous spirituality. They do not seek status; instead, it flows from the people. The sole goal of medicine, and the role of the healers, is to care of the mind, body and spirit of the people. There is no instance of Ao healers treating a patient and performing ceremonies for trade or a fee. They consider rituals and knowledge being used as a commodity for sale denudes traditional ideals and values. The traditional practice of offering a gift to healers, usually in the form of food or other practical items as a gesture of gratitude, is adequate. The central argument put forth rested on the notion of Ao traditional medicine as a sacred activity that cannot be bought or sold.

In the absence of any existing formal body of traditional medical knowledge and fixed criteria to distinguish a healer from the ordinary people, interestingly, it is never the case that one comes across a self-proclaimed healer (quack) who has abused and exploited traditional medical practices. Simply earned through his good conduct and selfless service towards the patient, his role in the Ao social and religious life as a healer is never looked at with suspicion or mistrust.

It is true that a *rachenlar* and his role were important in the socio-religious life of the Aos in ancient times as well as today to a great extent. He is not just a medicine man, healer or a

---

7. Gregory Cajete, in his book coined the term "ethnoscience," *Look to the Mountain* (2001).

shaman[8] but is one who plays a role which is much more significant, who combines in him the function of the augurer and performer of traditional rituals and sacrifices. A *rachenlar* who is endowed with certain divine powers is often seen playing an even higher role than a priest is, for a priest is a mere man of age who performs sacrifices for the people. Thus a true Ao healer is a person of incredible healing power, a "servant" of the suffering who uses his/her experience and insight into the human condition to treat and cure the afflicted.

Preliminary investigation discerned that traditional medicine of the Aos is vastly disintegrated and through colonial history has been hidden by people from church and government for fear of retribution or even imprisonment. The rationale was that it was devilish and against the Christian faith. In fact, the people's special knowledge of healing, which they gained through vision and experience and passed on through rituals, ceremonies and practices, was systematically stigmatized and suppressed by constructing the "healers" as quacks and the rituals as barbaric. The "stigmatization" of traditional medicine is critical since its essential philosophy is the belief system of the individual, and the individual's subsequent willingness to take responsibility for his or her own well-being.

The colonial idea of "traditional medicine" fell short of engaging the full vision of healers-patients identification of its richness and complexity by reducing it to the moment of interaction between healer and individual and a "treatment." On the other hand, the traditional medicine is seen by the Aos as a way of life and a collective dynamic. It is spiritual,

---

8. This is however, too general a term, to be used in this context.

expressed through land and ceremonies, and therefore holistic. Rather its foundation is understood as an ongoing healing journey of an individual in his pursuit in acquiring restoration and balance.

The pre-eminence on the external and material world results in a reduced sensitivity to the internal and spiritual, making physicians losing sense of the importance they play as a person in their interactions with their patients. In this regard, the knowledge of the healer's practice can help redirecting a physician's practice towards a more balanced approach, without necessitating physicians to learn completely new procedures, or communicate with the "spirits." Rather, the physician's personal self (the healer) can connect in "the human moment" (Hallowell, 1999) with the patient's personal self (the inner healer) in the hospital environment (the place) when both have a common understanding, or better say, a common belief system (the universal field).[9] Cumes describes a difference in our people: "The shaman embraces mystique rather than methodology, the compassionate and the emphatic rather than the objective and the impersonal, the intuitive rather than the rational. The marriage of science and shamanism creates equilibrium and fulfils the requirement of balancing the opposites for more complete healing." — (Cumes, 1999). Ultimately, the desired state (field) is an interpersonal relationship of trust and understanding.

References

Atran, Scott (1999), *"Managing the Maya Commons: The Value of Local Knowledge,"* (pp. 19-214), in V.D. Nazarea (ed.), *Ethno-Ecology: Situated Knowledge/Located Lives,* Tuscon: University of Arizona Press.

---

9. See Tom Janisse's *Healing Physicians: Physicians Healing.*

Battiste, Marie and Janes Youngblood Henderson (2000), *Protecting Indigenous Knowledge and Heritage: A Global Challenge*, Saskatoon, Saskatchewan: Purich Publishing Ltd.

Berlin, Brent and Elois Ann Berlin (1992), "Anthropological Issues in Medical Anthropology," in G. Prance (ed.) *Ethnobotany and the Search for New Drugs*. Ciba Foundation, Symposium publication, p. 185, Chiechester: Wiley.

Cajete, Gregory (1994), *Look to the Mountain: An Ecology of Indigenous Education*, Keyland, NC: Kivaki Press.

Cumes, D. (1999), *The Spirit of Healing*, Minnesota: Llewellyn Publications.

Hallowell, E. (1999), *The Value of the Human Moment in Medicine*, Group Practice Journal, October, Alexandria, VA: vol. 48, no. 9, American Medical Group Assocwiation.

Hammod-Tooke, David W. (1989), *Rituals and Medicines*, Johannesburg: Ad Donker Publisher.

Hufford, D.J. (1988), "Contemporary Folk Medicine," in N. Gevitz (ed.) *Other Healers: Unorthodox Medicine in the United States*, Baltimore: Johns Hopkins University Press.

Imchen, Panger (1993), *Ancient Ao Naga Religion and Culture*, New Delhi: Har-Anand Publications.

Kirscht, J.P. (1988), "The Health Belief Model and Predictions of Health Actions," in D.S. Gochman (ed.), *Health Behavior: Emerging Research Perspectives*, New York: Plenum.

Scott, C.J. (1997), "Ethnicity, Culture and the Delivery of Health-care Services: Enhancing System Outcomes in a Multicultural environment," in R. Rosen (ed.), *Emergency Medicine: Concepts and Clinical Practice*, St. Louis, MO: Mosby.

Sashinungla (2005), *Environment Preservation: A Philosophical Critique*, New Delhi: Decent Books, pp. 109-28.

Shiva, Vadana (2000), "Foreword: Cultural Diversity and the Politics of Knowledge," in George J. Dei, Budd L. Hall and Dorothy Goldin Rosenberg (ed.), *Indigenous Knowledge in Global Contexts*, Toronto: University of Toronto Press.

Stark, Rodney (1985), *The Sacred in a Secular Age*, Berkeley, CA: University of California Press.

Smith, Linda Tuhiwai (1999), *Decolonizing Methodologies Research and Indigenous Peoples,* London & New York: Zed Books Ltd.

World Health Organization, "Essential Drug and Medicine Policy, 21 August, 2001." www.who.int/medicines/organization/trm/orgtrmdef.shtml

Zysk, Kenneth G. (1993), *Religious Medicine: The History and Evolution of Indian Medicine,* New Brunswick and London: Transaction Publishers.

7

Caraka and the Notification of the Indian Medical Council on Physician-Patient Relationship
A Comparative Study

Ratna Dutta Sharma

THE present paper is an endeavour to make a comparative study of Caraka's view on physician-patient relationship with the nature of the said relation as has been stated or described in some of the relevant portions of the notifications made by the Medical Council of India published on 6th April, 2002 in part III, section 4 of the Gazette of India.

The entire paper is divided into three sections. In the first section some of the different aspects of the physician-patient relationship as conceived by Caraka are going to be dealt with. In the next section a few striking remarks made by Caraka are to be taken into consideration which seem to go against the nature of this relation as conceived by him. Is it possible to interpret these remarks so that the contradictions get resolved? In the concluding section specific portions of the said notifications made by the Medical Council of India are to be noted to see whether it is a continuation of Caraka's position, though capable of meeting the difficulties that his views have given rise to, through necessary modifications.

I

We often seek medical assistance from the physician known to be the health provider for the preservation and promotion of health. But the assistance sought may be successful if certain conditions stipulated by Caraka get fulfilled on the part of each of the factors involved, viz. (i) physician; (ii) patient; (iii) drug; and (iv) attendants.[1] It seems some reflections on the duties of the physician along with the specified conditions to be fulfilled by both the physicians and the patients for successful treatment will bring out the nature of the physician-patient relationship Caraka adhered to. The physician, according to Caraka, must aim at the well-being of the patient even though this may override other concerns — personal and others. The first condition which a physician is to satisfy is that he must have sound theoretical knowledge and practical experience regarding disease and medicine.[2] He must have acquaintance with the method of treatment provided by the different physicians. Caraka has given due emphasis on constant upgradation of the theoretical knowledge of the development of the medical science on the part of the physician.[3]

He has warned against the quacks who pretend themselves to be the expert physicians even though they fail to satisfy the required conditions. Their actual nature is to be exposed.[4] This

---

1. *Caraka Saṁhitā — Pūrba bhāgaḥ,* edited by Śrī Jayadevavidyalaṅkāra 2002, Motilal Banarasidas, Sūtrasthāna Navama Adhyāya, pp. 74-75.
2. *Caraka Saṁhitā* — vol. 2, edited by Kaviraj Brajendra Chandra Nag, Navapatra Prakashana, 1994 — Vimānasthāna, ch. viii, p. 137.
3. *Caraka Saṁhitā* — Ibid., p. 138.
4. *Caraka Saṁhitā* — vol. 1, edited by Kaviraj Brajendra Chandra Nag, Navapatra Prakashana, 1994, ch. x, p. 96.

indicates Caraka's vehement opposition to all types of pretentions. The physician, according to him, should be aware of the limits of his expertise and must have the sense of refusing the assignment which is beyond his capacity to handle.[5] He would never accept the charge of a patient even after being fully aware of the fact that the condition is totally out of his control, as that amounts to deception. Similarly the physician should avoid treating a man whom he ascertains to be free from disease. If he considers the disease of a patient to be curable and his treatment to be within his control, he must make honest use of his expertise for the benefit of the patient. But all these demand high moral quality of the patient. Morality, according to Caraka, consists in performing the acts prescribed by the scripture and which are conducive to the production of happiness.[6] Competence of a physician not only depends on having theoretical expertise and practical experience but also on living a moral life. Moral life, again, consists in living a disciplined and self-controlled life following the instructions of the scripture. By scripture, Caraka referred to the Vedas and those which do not contradict the Vedas.[7] The physician who is not only good in being life provider but also lives a moral life in the sense specified, is an ideal one in contrast to a good one whose attempt to treat the patient often leads to a success. An ideal physician must have a compassionate attitude towards the patient. He must be in a

---

5. *Caraka Saṁhitā* — vol. 1, edited by R.K. Sharma, Bhagwan Dash, Chowkhamba Sanskrit Series, Varanasi, 1999, Sūtrasthāna, ch. xi, p. 215.

6. *cikitsitastu saṁśrutya yo varṣamśratya mānajñaṣah nopakaroti vaidyāya naste tasyeha niṣkritiḥ*, 17, *Caraka Cintāmani* 1/4/55.

7. *Caraka Saṁhitā* — vol. II, edited by R.K. Sharma, Bhagwan Dash, Chowkhamba Sanskrit Series, Varanasi, 1999. Vimānasthāna, ch. viii, p. 221.

position to understand how the patients cope with their condition.

There is nothing to be surprised if a person takes such a physician as his friend, philosopher and guide. There is nothing to be surprised if the patient considers him to be the one who knows what is best for the patient. He may further accept that the physician has the right to take any decision in regard to his treatment. The physician may not disclose the actual position of the patient, the method of treatment he has adopted or is going to adopt in regard to his patient if the situation so demands. This would not surely violate the principle of truth which he is otherwise being instructed to adhere to.[8] According to Caraka it is incumbent on the patient to discharge his obligation towards the physician. He bitterly criticised the person who does not recompense the physician.[9] The physician, specifically the professional, may receive money, fame, etc. by rendering his service. But he must aim to make proper use of his expertise in the best interest of his patient. It is the duty of a patient to obey the instructions of the attending physician. Otherwise the very purpose of his approaching the physician would remain unfulfilled. Thus, Caraka included patient's adherence as the most essential condition to be satisfied for the success of treatment.

The personality of the physician, his outward appearance, must be such that he would make the patient feel comfortable to approach him. The physician, according to Caraka, should

---

8. *Caraka Saṁhitā* — vol. 1, edited by Kaviraj Brajendra Chandra Nag, 1994, Sūtrasthāna, ch. ix, p. 90.
9. *Çaraka Saṁhitā* — vol. I, edited by Prof. Priyavrat Sharma, Chawkhambha Orientalia, Varanasi, 1981, Vimānasthāna, ch. viii, p. 355.

not indulge in self-advertisement.[10] This he believes will cause annoyance in others and stand in the way of a comfortable relation between the physician and the patient. When the patient attains the position of having absolute confidence in the physician to the extent that the elements and aspects of their discussion will not get disclosed to a third party, then only he can share the confidential details of his own personality which might otherwise remain in suppression. This results in effective prognosis in the optimal interest of the patient. Since the patient puts his trust entirely on the physician, it is desired that he should make honest effort for keeping the interests of the patient.

In spite of all these, Caraka has instructed the physician to maintain a professional relation with the patient. Even though the physician is to have a deep concern for the patient, he must at the same time maintain an unemotional detachment also, otherwise it would be impossible for him to make use of the very painful and life-threatening therapy. The death of a patient under his treatment, for example, may make him too depressed to continue his profession. That Caraka was in favour of the physician keeping a distance from his patients becomes evident from his instruction to the physician to concentrate solely on the patient while paying a visit to the residence of the patient.[11] Perhaps this is the reason for his instruction to the physician to refuse the objects of enjoyment as gifts, specifically from the women. The physician is further advised not to treat a female in the absence of her husband. All these indicate that Caraka gave due emphasis on the physicians maintaining a distance from the women patients.[12]

---

10. Ibid.
11. Ibid.
12. Ibid.

Some of the questions initiated by Caraka's views as stated above can be construed thus:

1. The physician has been instructed to pay his sole attention to the patient. But it is quite conceivable that the interest of the patient may stand in conflict with the interest of society. In that case, what the physician should do?
2. The patient is an individual. As an individual he should have the right to know his own condition and to choose the method of treatment. The position that the physician knows what is best for the patient surely ignores the autonomy of the patient.
3. How far the principle of confidentiality is to be adhered to? If the physician's adherence leads to some unfavourable consequences, should he maintain it?
4. What would amount to the self-advertisement of the physician?

In the third section of this paper we will get the opportunity to refer to the relevant portions of the Notification of Indian Medical Association, March 2002 in order to have the plausible answers to these questions.

II

Caraka made certain assertions which appear to be in conflict with the nature of the relation between the physician and the patient as conceived by only himself. He instructed the physician not to treat the following persons:

1. One who considers himself to be a physician. In other words, the one who takes himself to be at par with the physician.

2. One who has no attendant.
3. A person who is not in a position to procure the elements necessary for treatment.
4. One who does not refute the charge brought against him.
5. A person who is terminally ill.
6. One who has lost all strength and vigour.
7. A person who is averse to the king.[13]
8 The unescorted lady.[14]

The honoured ideals of medical profession, according to Caraka, implies that the physician should aim at the physical well-being of the patient, even though this may override most other concerns including the personal one. This surely stands in direct conflict with the above-mentioned restrictions that Caraka himself had made.

Let us concentrate on the individual cases in the order in which they have been mentioned to find out the possible justification for those restrictions. One of the essential conditions which is to be fulfilled by the patient is that he must have complete trust and faith in the physician. This is what would prompt him to comply with the advice of the physician. But if he considers himself to be at par with the physician he may disobey the instruction of the physician. This may lead to the failure of the process of treatment undertaken

---

13. *Caraka Saṁhitā* — vol. II, Edited by R. K. Sharma, Bhagwan Dash, Chowkhamba Sanskrit Series, 2000, Vimānasthāna, ch. viii, p. 223.

14. *Caraka Saṁhitā* — vol. II, Edited by Kaviraj Brajendra Chandra Nag, Navapatra Prakashana, 1994, Vimānasthāna, ch. iii, p. 97.

and consequently give rise to the humiliating situation for the physician. Caraka's instruction may be interpreted as an attempt to make the physician aware of this situation.

Caraka had emphasised the role of the attendants in the execution of the instructions given by the physician. In the absence of the attendants, there will be difficulty in this respect which would make the process of treatment adopted ineffective. This surely constitutes a disgraceful situation for the physician. A physician must be cautious enough to avoid this situation. Caraka's instruction acknowledges the important role which the attendants play in the entire process of treatment.

Caraka opined that there is no necessity that each and every patient would be in a position to collect whatever is needed for the purpose of medication. On the other hand the possibility of the poor people being afflicted with complicated disease also cannot be ruled out. So the patient is to be treated by the appropriate method depending on his individual capacity. In the light of this, Caraka's instructions of not to treat a poor person may be taken to imply that expensive process of treatment should not be applied for such people.

One who fails to refute the charge brought against him is not eligible for receiving medical assistance, Caraka declared. This may be due to the fact that one of the grounds for being unable to refute the charge brought against a person may be his actual commission of the fault he is being charged of. Transgression of the instructions prescribed by the scriptures, according to Caraka, is the most heinous of all the crimes. Caraka's intention might be to resist the people from committing crimes. But one may fail to refute the charge brought against him on other grounds as well. He may not, for instance, have the capacity to argue in favour of his position.

Caraka has advised the physician not only to keep himself off from treating a patient of immoral character but also to maintain a safe distance from him. A physician is further instructed in the Notification of the Medical Council of India to expose without fear or favour, incompetent or corrupt, dishonest or unethical conduct on the part of the members of the profession. But how far it is practicable remains to be a question. He demanded high moral qualities both for the physician and the patient. In fact he gave utmost importance to the moral character of a human being.

The physician has been instructed by him not to provide medical assistance to the terminally ill patient and whose power of resistance has been diminished. This is quite consistent with the assertion he made elsewhere that the intelligent people always take preventive measures. They also seek the help of the physician at an early stage of the disease. The attempt to treat such patients in the end-stage often leads to failure. The chance of the humiliation of the attending physicians in those cases cannot be ruled out.

The reason for avoiding the treatment of a person who despises the king and who is despised by the king is not very difficult to understand. By treating a patient like him, a physician had to incur the wrath of the king. Caraka might have advised the physician to avoid such situations.

We have already mentioned that Caraka instructed the physician to keep safe distance from women. He insisted on the physician's maintaining certain restrictions while dealing with a female patient as has already been mentioned. According to him, a physician should not treat a lady in the absence of her guardian. The physician should not accept any gift item from the woman without the consent of her husband. Caraka, perhaps, has warned the physician of the severe consequences which he might have to face if he violates these restrictions.

From the above discussion, it follows that the existing situation might have prompted Caraka to make some of these restrictions. He has given some practical advice to the physicians so that he may not be driven to an unfavourable situation.

III

In this section we are going to concentrate on some specific portions of the Notification of Medical Council of India, March 2002, to see whether the position of Caraka in regard to the physician-patient relationship has remained constant. Let us first make an attempt to specify the common point of acceptance between the two. The principal objective of the medical profession is to serve the patient with full respect for the dignity of the profession. But this demands that he must be properly instructed in the art of healing. Reward or financial gain is to be treated as a subordinate consideration for a physician.[15] But the Notification of Medical Council of India 2002 declares that the responsibilities of the physician extend not only to the individual patient but also to society. According to Caraka, the physicians should merit the confidence of patients entrusted to their care. But the information about the patient and his surroundings confided by the patients to the physician, and defects in the disposition or character of patients should be revealed if the law of the state demands or if he himself feels it to be necessary for the greater interest. If the physician is aware that some patient is suffering from communicable, notifiable disease, it is considered to be his

15. *Caraka Saṁhitā* — vol. II, edited by Kaviraj Brajendra Chandra Nag, Navapatra Prakashana, 1994, *Vimānasthāna*, ch. viii, p. 137.

duty to inform the concerned public health authorities immediately[16]. This surely provides an answer to the question as to how far the principle of confidentiality is to be adhered to.

The Patient's Bill of Rights has accepted the right of the patient to obtain from his physician complete current information about his disease, treatment, etc. in terms the patient can be reasonably expected to understand. Not only that, the right of the patient to receive the information necessary to give informed consent before starting the procedure of treatment has also been recognized. The patient's right even to refuse the treatment and to be informed of the medical consequences of his action has been permitted.[17] So, the patient is no longer a silent receiver of the instructions of the physician who will always be ready to execute it. But his right to play an active role in the matter of his own treatment has been accepted. Still the question remains how far the patient is to be informed? It has been stipulated in the notification of the Medical Council of India that the physician should neither exaggerate nor minimize the gravity of a patient's condition. He should ensure himself that the patient, his relatives or his responsible friends have such knowledge of the patient's condition as will serve *the best interest of the patient*. If he thinks that the patient for instance is not to be informed of his actual position, as that would render his position further worse, he may not disclose it. Such measures can be justified on the ground of being able to serve the best interest of the patient.

---

16. *Caraka Saṁhitā* — vol. I, edited by Kaviraj Brajendra Chandra Nag, Navapatra Prakashana — 1994, Sūtrasthāna, ch. ii, p. 105.
17. Medical Council of India Notification, New Delhi, dated 11th March 2002, (published on 6th April 2002 in part III, section 4 of the Gazette of India)

Though Caraka instructed the physician not to indulge in self-advertisement, the question remained how far the physician is permitted to declare. Notification of The Medical Council of India, March 2002 declares, "A physician shall clearly display his fees and other charges on the board of his chamber and/ or the hospitals he is visiting, prescriptions should also by made clear if the physician himself dispensed any medicine." A physician is further advised to write his name and designation in full along with the registration particulars in his prescription letter-head. Printing of self-photograph or any such material of publicity on the letter-head or the signboard of the consulting room or any such clinical establishment is regarded as act of self-advertisement and unethical conduct on the part of the physician.[18]

Like Caraka, the present Notification also demanded high moral character for the physician. We have referred to the concept of morality Caraka adhered to. But the Notification of the Medical Council of India has mentioned a list of immoral activities of the physicians. This list includes among others — self-advertising, exploitation of patients, offering and receiving gifts, gratuity and commission in return for referring, recommending or procuring for any patient medical, surgical or any other treatment, solicitation of the patient, etc. Instead of prohibiting a physician to treat an unescorted lady, the present Notification has explicitly stated, "Abuse of professional position by committing adultery or improper conduct with a patient or by maintaining an improper association with a patient, will render a physician liable for disciplinary action as provided under the Indian Medical Council Act, 1956 or the concerned State Medical Council Act."[19]

18. Ibid.

19. Ibid.

All these show that the main contention of Caraka has been kept unaltered even in the recent Notification of the Medical Council of India 2002. But attempts have been made to remove the difficulties associated with Caraka's position through different stipulations and clarifications. The further point to note is that it has been specifically mentioned that no physician should arbitrarily refuse treatment to a patient. The only situation when a physician can refuse treatment is when the patient is suffering from an ailment which is not within the range of experience of the physician. But we have taken note of the specific instructions of Caraka which were, to a large extent, the outcome of the existing social condition. Such conditions being changed, these restrictions have lost relevance and consequently been dropped out. After making explicit declaration that the physician must give priority to the interest of the patients, Caraka as a physician was very much concerned about the honour or position of the physician in society. He has given some practical advice to the physician so that he can avoid the humiliating situation. The ground offered by Caraka for instructing the physician not to provide medical assistance to the patient under certain conditions, I presume, goes against the ideal of universal service to humanity.

We have mentioned that Caraka has stipulated how a physician should behave specifically with the ladies. But in the Notification of the Medical Council of India there is no such specification. The patient here has been considered as a patient wihout any gender/sex categorization. This indicates that the outlook has been changed altogether. The relevant stipulations have been made in the broad sense so that it applies to the patient as such irrespective of his/her economic, social, political status and other considerations as have already been mentioned.

8

Non-Reason, Madness, Mental Health Science and the Ethics of Psychoanalysis

Anup Kumar Dhar
Ranjita Biswas

> . . . ethics cannot be put into words . . .
> — Wittgenstein, 1961: 6.421

THIS work looks at the relation of "non-Reason" and the institution of "mental health science." To look at the relation it asks a few questions: Does non-Reason get reduced to "madness" in the institution of mental health science? Is the category of madness conjured up to repress/foreclose non-Reason from the domain of the possible? Does the institution of mental health science *only* rein in minds? Does it *not* try to understand minds? Does it attend to the complex vicissitudes of the mind *only* through Reason, only through what passes off *as* Reason? Does it attend to non-Reason only through hegemonic understandings of reason, through what we could provisionally represent *as* Reason (reason with a capital "R")? Does it work *only* towards what has emerged in a given socio-cultural formation as *hegemonic* reason, *as* Reason? Does it rein in minds by turning away from non-Reason? Does the whole of the institution of mental health science *turn away* from non-

Reason? Or do certain moments in the larger canvas of mental health science attend to non-Reason? Are those moments — moments that *turn to* non-Reason — related in ways more than one to psychoanalysis; more precisely, to a particular rendition and understanding of psychoanalysis? To think through some such questions we take as representative a statement in Bengali made by a "mentally distressed patient" — a statement that in a way puts down the "feeling" of the recipient of mental health care —

> *āpnara śudhu monke bāndhte jānen, monke bujhte paren na.*
>
> (all you psychiatrists know is how to *rein in* minds; you don't *understand* the mind.)

The above is a statement made by a "patient" in a psychiatric hospital. The "patient" whom we cannot name due to a certain code of confidentiality had been under a long period of treatment in the same psychiatric hospital. Every time the "patient" was called for an interview with the psychiatrist, she came with a small notebook. The notebook contained pages of "incoherent" ramblings from which she would try to read out excerpts for us. Each time the "patient" made a demonstration of her "madness" in an *explicit* manner, the number and dose of medicines increased. In the subsequent sessions the "patient" appeared more groggy and slurred. But every time the "patient" looked capable of continuing her (broken) dialogue with the psychiatrist . . . continue the dialogue in the hope of establishing her sanity. Until, finally, somewhat in exasperation the "patient" made the above statement. The above statement comes as a certain eruption of truth; it is as if the truth was thrown up at the institution by a harassed "victim" of the institution — the truth thrown up by a victim from behind the bars. How would the institution of science in general and the institution of mental health science in particular attend to this aspersion? What would the psychiatrist do? How would "He" respond to the charge?

The doctor-patient relation (here the relation between the "psychiatrist" and the "mentally ill" or the more fashionable "mentally challenged") has been an area of intense debate, discussion and speculation. The doctor has been described as the *expert*, godlike or godsend, who bestows health or life. The patient is said to be a *layperson*, who entrusts faith, belief and the authority in the doctor to make decisions and judgments on his/her behalf.

It is the patient's right to expect reasonable skill and care from the doctor in an effort to get relief. This entails unconditional attention to the patient's suffering and welfare as well as judicious use of the doctor's knowledge and expertise. The patient is also entitled to all information pertaining to the illness, its nature, course, prognosis, treatment undertaken, its consequences and hazards and also reserves the right to refuse treatment at any point of time. Assuming the doctor to be the expert, the autonomy of the patient is as much important.

The doctor is bound by the Hippocratic oath and he not only bears the moral responsibility to do no harm but also provides health benefits to the patient. The medical profession itself is said to be self-regulatory, bound by a code of medical ethics that defines the duties of the doctor towards the patient, duties that bear an intimate relation to the patient's rights and expectations. In this respect medical ethics is not merely a moral parameter, it is also a legally sanctioned code of conduct. Medical ethics as it is understood commonly could be made to derive from two different understandings of the doctor-patient relationship — Kaplan & Saddock, 1994: pp. 1189-90:

1. *Medical Paternalism;* and
2. *Autonomy Theory.*

Medical Paternalism is the traditional model for the physician-patient relationship, where the doctor is supposed to treat the patient as a caring parent would treat a young child. The physician is presumed to know what is best for the patient just as a parent/father would for the (girl) child and has no obligation to explain each decision or to ask permission to perform actions that are done to benefit the patient. The physician is presumed to *have* knowledge that the patient may be very nearly incapable of understanding or, in the physician's judgement, is better off not knowing. The "infantilism"–"non-Reason"–"immaturity" connection is presumed in this model.

On the other hand the ***Autonomy Theory***[1] conceives of the relationship between the doctor and the (adult) patient as that between two responsible persons — responsible for their own and separate selves. In this approach the patient is presumed to have the ability and the right to make rational and responsible life decisions. The patient is autonomous (self-governing) and has right to self-determination that must be respected even if the best-intended decisions are thought to be against the patient's best interests.

Because of the unique nature of the sufferings of the mentally ill, the principles of beneficence and autonomy may

---

1. Autonomy theory also holds that paternalistic treatment may be justified when those persons lack the capacity to be autonomous — for example children, profoundly retarded persons and sometimes persons branded psychotic. The author of this paper remains justifiably disappointed by this giving up on the principle of autonomy, by this *turning away* from the principle of autonomy by the very theorists and proponents of autonomy.

be interpreted in conflicting ways giving rise to conflicts in value and beliefs about appropriate "care-healing-cure." While many proponents of informed consent feel this is a moral condition underscoring all doctor-patient relationships, it obviously poses significant problems when applied to the mentally ill. The notion of consent is a debated virtue when it concerns the mentally ill who could also be considered purportedly *irrational, sub-human,* a theme that keeps recurring in all areas of their life and not just in their treatment. The basic question is thought to be whether a "mentally ill" person is capable of giving informed consent, given the state of impaired reasoning and suspended ability to make rational choices.

Critics of the school of informed consent argue that mentally ill patients are not always capable of giving informed consent for the appropriate mode of treatment. They maintain that to make informed consent a right by statute, while desirable in an ethical sense, would only hinder the ability of patients to receive the treatment they need. Many psychiatrists argue strongly for compulsive treatment on the grounds that a patient's right to treatment necessitates a reciprocal obligation by psychiatrists to provide the most effective and humane treatment possible, even against the patient's expressed wishes. They argue that a psychiatrist is in a much better position than either the patient or the courts to assess the treatment needed and decide what is best for a particular patient. Furthermore, they contend that the excessive legal regulation of treatment procedures clearly subordinates the treatment of mental illness to "a never-ending series of adversarial confrontations" between patients and doctors. Another dimension to the issue of consent is whether an involuntarily confined person (a number of psychiatric "cases" need institutional treatment at some time or other, during the course of their illness), whose overriding concern is to leave the institution, can give "free voluntary" consent to treatment. In most cases, the subtle and not-so-subtle pressures of the attending psychiatrists, given his/her virtue of knowing what is *wrong with them* and what is *right for them,* the family and/or the community and given their overtly altruistic concerns, render the "consent" less voluntary — and in some cases involuntary. This is particularly important if a patient is given to believe that his or her release is contingent upon cooperation with treatment which in most cases boils down to complying with the orders without questioning and therefore making a show of "good behavior." "Parole" is a system by which patients who are well after a period of institutional treatment can go home for a short visit. Their behaviour during this short stay at home then becomes the basis for further discharge plans. The question that often arises in this context: Is involuntary confinement a way to protect individuals from the potential consequences of their illness or is it a form of *social control* and *surveillance*?[2]

It appears from such arguments that the basic conditions for informed consent — adequate access to information, ability to receive, understand and interpret information, freedom from both overt and covert coercion in making and executing decisions (say in giving consent) — perhaps do not apply to those individuals designated "mentally ill." One line of

---

2. In this context, it would be important to put rather sharply the question of the particular positioning of psychiatry? What is psychiatry's position in the larger canvas of medicine? What is the role-goal-aim of psychiatry? Is it an apparatus of "social control" and "surveillance"? Is it an appendage of the State? Or is it an apparatus of "care-healing-cure"?

contention that could follow from this: the psychiatric institution is the best refuge for the mentally ill; the psychiatrist is the best arbiter of what is good and what is bad for the patient. The other related line of contention could be that if these people are thought to be incapable of informed consent, if they are thought to be incapable of making "rational" and "autonomous" choices, if they *lack in rational capabilities*, can we then at all make an argument for the "rights of the mentally ill?"

While one could make an argument for rights of all "sane" individuals, of all "conscious," rational, choosing subjects, of all "normal" minds, one could not make an argument for the rights of the "insane," the "mad," the "non-conscious," the "abnormal" among minds. The argument for the rights of the "mad human" (the *mad* human is perhaps *less than human*) appears furthermore thin in the case of the "mad woman." It is thinner still in the case of the "mad non-white woman," the "woman" and the "colonial" being further repositories of non-Reason, non-Reason understood as "madness" in the psychiatric institution.

The somewhat converse argument (an argument I would wish to pursue) could be that this distinction (a distinction, or difference that borders on a certain *dualism*) — this distinction between the normal, the ordered mind and the abnormal, the deranged mind — flows out of a certain hegemony of Reason over the *others* of reason, which in turn, flows perhaps from our allegiance to Aristotle's "Laws of thought" or from our belief in "Classical two-valued logic."

From the rather simple question of "institutional access" — access of the "mentally ill" to cure-care (which in actuality is a question of health-related infrastructures, say the number of beds, the number of medical and paramedical staff per patient, etc.) — from the question of the *humane* treatment of the "mentally ill" (which in actuality is a question of *not* the quantity but the *quality* of health care available) we move over to the question of knowledge — to a certain violence of knowing and an ethics of knowing. This brings us to the question of the relation of *reason* to *non-Reason;* the pathologization of non-Reason *vis-à-vis* Cartesian Reason; the re-writing of non-Reason as *madness* would therefore come up for discussion (even if somewhat tangentially) in this work. We would have to ask whether reason's relation to non-Reason takes off first from a certain "knowledge of the mind"; knowledge of the mind, *in general?* Does it then find itself refracted into a certain "knowledge of the normal mind" and thereafter into a "knowledge of the abnormal mind," the "abnormal mind" being the "mind of non-Reason," or for that matter, of the "mind of madness," the mind of madness being very nearly "no mind" at all? Is it then also a question of the "mind" knowing the "no-mind," the "non-mind?" Is it then a question of "reason" knowing "non-Reason"; "science" knowing "madness?" Is it then also a question of "western science" knowing "savage non-Reason," "male reason" knowing "woman's madness"? Does the knowledge of non-Reason, non-Reason understood *as* madness, find itself refracted further into a "knowledge of the colonial woman's madness" or for that matter into a certain "knowledge of the mad colonial woman," the "colonial" and the "woman" being further repositories of non-Reason, non-Reason understood as madness?

We thus find the world of "mental health science" breaking down into *two* — mind/non-mind, normal mind/abnormal mind, white male reason/native woman's non-Reason, sanity/madness, order/breakdown — which is never really *two,* which in actuality is *one,* which in actuality is the logic of the *One* and the *Same.* This is because *non-Reason,* or for that matter, non-Reason understood as *madness,* is not another, is not an Other, but is simply the negative, the dark, the derogatory, the *lacking* underside of Reason. In this particular thought world, madness is the "constitutive inside" of hegemonic reason while non-Reason is the "constitutive outside."

Thus to think of an ethical relation in the mental health clinic one perhaps needs to look at the hegemony of Reason ("p") over non-Reason ("non-p") — at the very reduction of non-Reason to madness (to *lacking* p) — to its *being* pathological by virtue of its being non-Reason, i.e. by virtue of its being not-reason (not-p). There can perhaps be no question of the "rights of the mad" without the concomitant question of an ethical relation (notwithstanding the impossibility that haunts any such relation) of Reason/Science/Doctor with non-Reason/madness/patient. An ethical relation between doctor and patient is not just a question of the humane or the sensitive handling of the patient by the doctor. It is also a question of the presuppositions, of the conceptual apparatus that drives the mental health professional to engage with the patient in the way he or she engages now. In other words, one needs to look at the structures of knowledge/reasoning that inform the response of the "courier of scientific knowledge" (Achuthan, 2004) in the mental health clinic. An ethical relation in the mental health clinic thus relates as well to an *ethics of knowing;* it relates to the way one knows, what one knows, how one knows, what results from such knowing. Is there a certain objectification of the "known" in the process of knowing? Is the process in one way or the other somewhat reductionist? Does the "knower" homogenize the "known" in the process? Does "knowing" in any way reduce the "known" to silence; is there a certain exclusion . . . a *foreclosure*?

The other more fundamental problem regarding any knowledge/science/discourse concerning "madness," or for that matter, concerning any "history of madness" is that the whole field is fraught with a few nearly insurmountable epistemological difficulties: Is there any witnessing to madness? Who can witness or rather who *can* lay claim to witnessing madness, to witnessing the singular and irreducible alterity of *the* (singular) Other? The very same difficulties would perhaps haunt the possibility of any "knowledge of the mind." Who knows? Who knows whom? How do we know? Do we know through our minds? How then does one mind know another? What are the bases of our claims to knowledge? Are our claims tied in one way or the other to history/culture? Here we are "echoing and engaging with Kant's "what can I know?" and his probing of the limits of reason and reason as a limit" — Didur and Heffernan, 2003:2.

Foucault writes a *history of knowing,* which in other words, is a *history of silencing,* the *silencing of non-Reason.* He writes a history of *knowing/silencing non-Reason,* he writes a history of *Reason knowing/silencing non-Reason.* He writes, in the process, a history of non-Reason, which in other words, is *also* a history of silence. He shows through his history (or in other words, his story) how the history of non-Reason (as well as of Reason) is in reality the history of the hegemony of Reason over non-Reason. Foucault shows how in the process of knowing there is a certain play of power; how a history of knowing is in reality a history of the exclusion of non-Reason from thought itself — of the *reduction of non-Reason to madness* — where madness is the constitutive inside of hegemonic Reason and non-Reason is the constitutive outside of hegemonic Reason. Foucault wants therefore to re-write a history of "non-Reason/madness" itself . . . before being captured . . . "and paralyzed in the nets of classical reason." He wants "non-Reason/madness" to be the *subject* of his book in every sense of the word: its theme and its first-person narrator, its author, madness speaking about itself . . . madness speaking on the basis of its own experience and under its own authority, and *not* from within the language of reason. Foucault wants to write a *history of silence.* Derrida (1978) points at the very impossibility of Foucault's *archaeology of silence:* "is there a history of silence? . . . is not an archaeology, even of silence, a logic, that is, an organized language, a project, an order, a syntax, a work?" Derrida asks: Do we not access madness with the language of the very "reason" we denounce? Does not our verdict unceasingly reiterate the crime? Foucault, of course, is *not* unaware of the near unconscious complicity with the language of reason that haunts his project — his project at accessing non-Reason before the *Decision.* But then, Foucault pursues a project that is impossible. It is as if an ethico-politics of the (im)possible — ethics as the "experience of the impossible." Otherwise we would only be "continuing the Cartesian exclusion" of non-Reason by *Reason.* Derrida, instead, stresses the *moment* of non-Reason that inheres inalienably *in* reason — non-Reason as a possible menace at the very heart of the intelligible. Derrida prefers *dissension* instead of *Decision* — the single act that separates reason and madness. *Dissension* underlines instead "a self-dividing action, a cleavage and torment interior to meaning *in general,* a division within the very act . . . *dissension* is internal. The exterior (is) the interior . . ." (Derrida, 1978). Derrida, while never subscribing to the Foucauldian notion of *Decision,* reads in the history of "mental health science" the history of a *return* (Derrida, 1994) — a *return* to the self-dividing action — to the cleavage and torment interior to meaning *in general,* which in other words, is also the symptomatic return of the repressed.

Hence the possibility of a *return* to *non-Reason. A return of Freud* — a return *of* Freud *to* "non-Reason" at the level of its *language.* For Freud *too* non-Reason would be madness, but this time one would resume a *dialogue with non-Reason* and lift, as if, the Cartesian interdiction. And lift it as if to reopen for a moment a dialogue that was broken off once in the classical age and that would be broken off again by the language of psychological positivism. Psychology *breaks off* from non-Reason, from a certain "truth" of non-Reason. Psychoanalysis *breaks off* from psychology by speaking with the non-Reason that speaks within Reason such that Reason is always already under erasure. But that too, only for a moment — operating as only a *hinge* (Derrida, 1994) in this nearly unsuspended history of suspended dialogue.

> Freud, *returns to non-Reason* (Derrida, 1994).
> Lacan (1977a, 1977b) and Derrida (1978, 1987, 1994), in, albeit contradictory ways *returns to Freud.*

Davidson returns not to Freud but to the history of psychoanalysis. For Davidson the history of psychoanalysis (as of any history of nearly any science) is premised not around the biography of a historical figure (here Freud) nor around the mere diachronic unfolding of events *but* around the history of "structurally related system of concepts," around the "conceptual space, that lies below, or behind, the work of any particular author." To write a history of psychoanalysis one will perhaps have to look at "whether the structure of concepts associated with Freud's writing continues, extends, diverges from, or undermines the conceptual space of nineteenth-century psychiatry." One needs to write an account of the concepts used in psychoanalysis — an account of their historical origins and transformations, their rules of combination, and their employment in a mode or "style of reasoning." This task presumes that one can isolate the distinctive features of nineteenth century psychiatry and articulate their rules of combination. One must then look whether Freud's conceptual space is a continuation or a break with that of his predecessors.

One moment in Freud's conceptual space that marks a break with that of his predecessors is related to the question of his return to non-Reason as also to his setting-up of a dialogue with non-Reason (the other moments are related to his *return* to the question of "women/sexual difference" and "native/ colonial difference.") This return of a *certain* Freud or of a *certain* strain (even if marginal) of psychoanalysis to non-Reason at the level of language — this setting-up of a dialogue with non-Reason — a certain standing *face to face* with non-Reason is fundamental to any ethical relation, to any relation based on responsibility[3] in the mental health clinic.[4]

Ethics of Knowing

To think of *knowing* . . . to think of a possible *ethics of knowing* . . . a knowing that is epistemologically less violent . . . a knowing that is not a silencing . . . as also to think of the impossibility that haunts any knowing . . . one perhaps needs

---

3. "In her work "Righting Wrongs" — delivered at Oxford University as part of an Amnesty International series of lectures "Human Rights and Human Wrongs" — Spivak describes two forms of culture — responsibility-based (subaltern) and rights-based (Northern) — arguing both need supplementation, one by the other . . ." . (Didur and Heffernan, 2003:7).

4. One can explore the *possibilities inhering in such a possible return to non-Reason* in the context of Lacanian psychoanalysis. One can, along with Lacan, delineate the contours of an ethical engagement with non-Reason — an engagement that is also an engagement with the phenomenology of mental dis-*ease* — an engagement that tries at the same time to be epistemologically less violent.

to move away from the prevailing "ethical ideology" (Badiou, 2001). The prevailing "ethical ideology" has two "philosophical poles." First, a (vaguely Kantian) universalizing pole which, indifferent to the particularity of any given situation, proscribes in any advance any possibility of an organized . . . *situated* intervention in the name of collective "Good": ethics here is grounded in the abstract universality of general "human" attributes or rights. And, second, a (vaguely Levinasian) differential pole, attuned to the irreducible alterity of the Other: ethics here is expressed in an equally abstract respect for mainly cultural differences. Neither *this* universality nor *this* alterity, Badiou suggests, can be rigorously founded without tacit reference to theology; either way, the [prevailing] ethical ideology conceives of "[wo]man" as a fundamentally passive, fragile and *mortal* entity — as a potential victim to be protected (most often, as a "marginalized," "excluded" or "Third World" victim) by a dutiful, efficient, and invariably "Western" benefactor/exploiter.

Badiou "rejects the almost universally accepted argument that ethics should essentially concern the Other as such (as potential victim of violence or misrecognition) . . . Perhaps nothing is more orthodox today than a generalized reverence for the other *qua* other . . . [the other (every other) is indeed *other,* absolutely other: *Tout autre est tout autre* . . . the other as alterity] . . . the alterity of the other . . . Couched most notably in terms of the logic of the *gift,* Derrida's ethical reflections circle obsessively around notions of inaccessibility and secrecy, around that which is beyond [re]presentation or identification, around subjective impossibility, around "madness" and "forgetting" . . ." (Badiou, 2001: xv-xxiv). Badiou tries to provide an "inspiring, rigorously argued alternative to the tired moralizing truisms of neo-Kantian universalism on the one hand [along with its more American offshoot: liberal analytic jurisprudence] and a more or less tolerant liberal communitarianism on the other" (Badiou, 2001: xxx).

> [Badiou's] *ethic of* [subjective[5]] *truths* presumes that every individual can be active and . . . is indifferent to established or state-sanctioned differences, operates in the realm of practical division (for or against the event[6]), and situates its affirmation precisely there where the stay of the situation can see only the non-known and the non-obvious. (Badiou, 2001: italics mine).

This journey from the prevailing/hegemonic "ethical ideology" to Badiou is also a (not too explicit) journey from classical philosophy *to* a "psychoanalytically inspired" philosophy (Lecan, 1990: 7). It is a journey from the "philosophy of the Cogito" to a philosophy that puts the Cogito under erasure. It is a journey from a "philosophy of presence" to a "philosophy-of-presence-put-*under-erasure*." One could ask: why do we need to make this journey from philosophy (epistemology — as an encounter with knowledge) to psychoanalysis (analysis is an encounter with *non-Reason* — with *madness*)? Is it because "psychoanalysis renders visible the constitutive *madness* of modern philosophy"? Is it because psychoanalysis brings to the foreground what was foreclosed in the Cartesian theatre? And this is precisely "what Lacan was

5. "Access to the realm of truth . . . is wholly subjective: It is founded only on the subjects who "bear" its trajectory." (Badiou, 2001: ix).

6. " . . . a truth procedure can begin only with some sort of break with the *ordinary situation* in which it takes place — what Badiou calls an *event*. An event has no objective or verifiable content. Its "happening" cannot be proved, only affirmed and procailmed." (Badiou, 2001:ix).

doing all the time: reading hysteria or obsessional neurosis as a philosophical "attitude of thought towards realtiy" (the obsessional compulsion to think — "if I stop thinking, I will cease to exist" as the truth of the Cartesian *cogito ergo sum*) . . ." — Zizek, 1998:2.

> . . . the whole of modern philosophy, from Descartes onward, involves an inherent reference to the threat of madness, and is thus a desperate attempt to draw a clear line that separates the transcendental philosopher from the madman (Descartes: how do I know I'm not hallucinating reality?; Kant: how to delimit metaphysical speculation from . . . hallucinatory rambling?). — Zizek, 1998:2.

The question that we wish to ask in this work: Can psychoanalysis set up a meaningful engagement with non-Reason and *not* reduce non-Reason to *mere* madness? Or more precisely, can the (Lacanian) analytic setting offer a possible conceptual space to explore questions of *othering* (*othering* that flows not from the overt violence of and in the mental health institution but also flows from hegemonic forms of knowing) as well as explore questions related to *an other heading* (Derrida, 1992) — *an other heading* of *classical epistemology* — *an other heading of the classical clinical encounter* . . . such that there is an engagement with non-Reason . . . such that there is no turning away from non-Reason? It is in answer to this question that one can bring up the somewhat representative example of Lacanian psychoanalysis. This is of course not to say that we propose to turn every mentally distressed person to Lacanian psychoanalysis. We wish Lacanian psychoanalytic setting (with reference to an *ethics of the real* [Chakrabarti and Dhar, 2002]) to be an ethical bind on all clinical settings in the mental health situation. The setting of Lacanian psychoanalysis is, therefore, used and reiterated to bring up and highlight the idea/ideal of a clinical engagement we wish to imagine — how while not giving up on an engagement with the irreducible phenomenology of mental disease/distress one could still think of a clinical engagement — a listening to and a "speaking with" (Moitra, 2002) — how one could still think of a possible relationship with non-Reason that could be ethical not just at the level of institutional practice but even at the level of knowledge/truth production.

References

Achuthan, A. (2004), "Women and Midwifery in the Indian Context: Between the Practical and the Propositional" in *Women's Education and the Politics of Gender,* Kolkata: Behune College.

Badiou, A. (2001), *Ethics: An Essay on the Understanding of Evil* — translated and introduced by Peter Hallward, London: Verso.

Chakrabarti, A. and A. Dhar, (2002), "The Nodal Possibility of Entry Point: Theorizing the End of Capitalism" paper for conference "Subjects of Economy" organized by the Association for Economic and Social Analysis and Rethinking Marxism.

Davidson, A.I., (2001), *The Emergence of Sexuality: Historical Epistemology and the Formation of Concepts,* Harvard University Press.

Derrida, J., (1978), *Writing and Difference,* Routledge and Kegan Paul.

———, (1987), *The Post Card: From Socrates to Freud and Beyond,* Trans. Alan Bass, University of Chicago Press.

———, (1992), *The Other Heading: Reflections on Today's Europe,* Indiana University Press.

———, (1994), "To Do Justice to Freud: The History of Madness in the Age of Psychoanalysis," *Critical Inquiry,* 20 (Winter 1994).

Dhanda, Amita, (2000), *Legal Order and Mental Disorder,* Sage.

Foucault, Michel, (1988), *Madness And Civilization: A History of Insanity in the Age of Reason,* Vintage.

Kaplan, H.I. Saddock, J.A. Grebb (ed.) (1994), *Synopsis of Psychiatry,* 7th edn., New Delhi: B.I. Waverly Pvt. Ltd.

Lacan, J. (1977a), *Ecrits,* Tavistock.

——— (1977b), *The Four Fundamental Concepts of Psychoanalysis*, Hogarth Press.

Moitra, S. (2002), *Feminist Thought: Androcentrisim, Communication and Objectivity*, New Delhi: Munshiram Manoharlal.

Plumwood, V. (1993), *Feminism and the Mastery of Nature*, Routledge.

Zizek, S. (1994), *The Sublime Object of Ideology*, Verso.

——— (1988), "Introduction: Cogito as a Shibboleth" in S. Zizek (ed.), *Cogito and the Unconscious*, Durham: Duke University Press.

9

Shades of Confidentiality in Physician-Patient Relationship

In the Context of Mental Health

Somdatta Bhattacharyya

PHYSICIAN-patient relationship is a very significant issue in medical ethics, and for the last 1500 years the sanctity of communication between doctor-patient has been valued very much. In the core values for the medical profession BMA 1995, we observe that the patient-doctor relationship should be a partnership of mutual trust with the personal consultation remaining the bedrock of the medical practice. Such doctor-patient relationship has come under some serious scrutiny in ethical debates over issues, such as withholding confidential information, obtaining informed consent, boundary transgression and so on. Some of these issues arise from the physician's end and some of them from the patient's end, irrespective of the fact that all of them are important for establishing such physician-patient bond. In this paper the main focus will be on one such ethical issue, just mentioned, i.e. the concept of confidentiality with which all physicians are concerned, especially those who are related to mental health. Here the problem of confidentiality would be addressed in the context of mental health only, precisely speaking, in the context of psychotherapy.

But before going to that problem of confidentiality in psychotherapy, first I would like to analyse the nature of physician-patient relationship in the context of psychotherapy. Now, it is more or less an accepted fact that relationship or interconnectedness between two people has been significant in all healing from the period of Hippocrates and Galen. Relationship can be defined as "the state of being related, a condition or character based on this kinship."[1] Again from another end, it is quite interesting to observe famous existentialist Boss's opinion that all illnesses and treatments are developed out of the patient's disturbed human relationships.[2] However, in this discussion, an elucidation will be given of a special kind of relationship or betweenness of people, viz. physician-patient relationship in the context of psychotherapy.

To talk about psychotherapeutic relationship, we cannot altogether eliminate the common knowledge that ordinary human relationship can have therapeutic value. The old structures of religion, accepted moral order and extended family networks used to provide supportive relationships and healing matrices for many people. There is a possibility that psychotherapy as an institutionalised profession became necessary as a consequence of such a decline in the society and quality of healing relationships,which were available in previous centuries. This view can be debated. Of course other alternative causes can be observed for emergence of psychotherapy as a profession. But that is a different issue altogether.

---

1. C. T. Onions (1973) *The Shorter Oxford English Dictionary: On Historical Principles*, vol. 2, Oxford Clarendon Press.
2. M. Boss (1963), *Psychoanalysis and Daseinanalysis* (L.B. Lfefre, trans.), New York: Basic Books.

Now leaving behind the common knowledge, from the technical point of view, it is generally held that the pivot of psychotherapy is the therapeutic relationship, which differs from all other professional relationships. This kind of therapeutic relationship between clinician and patient/client has got a special and unique nature. According to T. Byram Karasu, some new as well as old and enduring ethical dilemmas in the practice of psychotherapy may be derived from this unique relationship.[3] Thus some ethical problems, however, affect psychotherapeutic practice that differs in shade and degree from other branches of medicine. The problem of confidentiality is one such problem, which has got a unique nature in psychotherapy than in any other branch of medicine. It can be said that the unusual emotional bond that developed between therapists and patients/clients lies at the root of these differences. It has been compared to that of a parent and a child and is unlike other professional or contractual relationships, such as teacher to student, clergy to parishioner, or lawyer to client (Gabbard, 1989).[4] It is distinct not only in the intimacies of personal life, emotions that are revealed, but due to deep-seated dependency, attraction and affection, that are often aroused.

Here it should be mentioned that there are different psychotherapy systems and it is not very easy to demonstrate clear advantages differentially attributable to different psychotherapy systems. But there is a common consensus of agreement among all of them regarding the crucial importance

---

3. T.B. Karasu, "Ethical Issues in Psychotherapy Practice," p. 320, *An Introduction to the Psychotherapies*, ed. by Sidney Bloch, Oxford Medical Publications, Oxford University Press, 3rd edn., 1996.
4. G.O. Gabbard (ed.) (1989), *Sexual Exploitation in Professional Relationships*, American Psychiatric Press. Washington DC.

of therapeutic relationship. Researchers like Frank (1979) and Hynan (1981) observed that the client, the psychotherapist and the therapeutic relationship between them are repeatedly more closely related to outcome than whatever technique has been used.[5]

Regarding therapeutic relationship and the factors, which are important and responsible for establishing and maintaining such relationship, Kahn opined that — "Most beginning clinicians understand that it is important to live by the basic ground rules of therapy. Confidentiality must be honoured and the boundaries of therapeutic relationship must be respected, which means remembering every moment that our clients are neither friends nor lovers. Most therapists know these rules, but until one has grasped just how subtle and complex the relationship can be, and how important the therapist becomes to the client, one is likely to seriously underestimate how easy it is to damage the therapy. The slightest breach of confidentiality can be magnified by the client into a major betrayal; a chance encounter with a client outside the consulting room can evolve into a problematic social situation and have serious repercussions."[6]

Petruska Clarkson in his book "*The Psychotherapeutic Relationship*," mentions that Kahn introduces a perspective on using the relationship as a central factor in all of

---

5. a) J.D. Frank (1979), "The Present Status of Outcome Studies," *Journal of Consulting and Clinical Psychology* 47:310-16.

   b) M.T. Hynan (1981), On the advantages of assuming that the techniques of psychotherapy **are/**, *Psychotherapy: Theory, Research and Practice.* 18:11-3.

6. M.D. Kahn (1991), *Between the Therapist and Client: The New Relationship,* New York: W.H. Freeman.

psychotherapy. According to him, the relationship is the therapy.[7]

If indeed the therapeutic relationship is one of the most, if not the most, important factor in successful psychotherapy, one would expect much of the training in psychotherapy to be training in the intentional use of relationship. Some psychotherapists claim that psychotherapy requires use of only one kind of relationship, or at the most two. Some specifically exclude the use of certain kinds of relationship. For example, Goulding and Goulding(1979),[8] in transactional analysis, minimize the use of transference, whereas Moiso (1985),[9] also in transactional analysis, sees it as a central focal point of classical Bernian psychotherapy. Gestaltists Polster and Polster (1973)[10] and the existentialist May (1969)[11] focus on the existential nature of the therapeutic relationship. But in the history of psychotherapy, a different voice can be found in some psychotherapeutic approaches. They pay hardly any theoretical attention to the nature of the relationship and they may attempt to be entirely free of content. For example, in some approaches to hypnotherapy or Neuro-Linguistic Programming (NLP), therapeutic changes are claimed to be made by the patient without the practitioner necessarily knowing what these changes may be. But again psychoanalysts,

---

7. Clarkson Petruska, *"The Psychotherapeutic Relationship."*
8. M.M. Goulding and R.L. Goulding (1979), *Changing Lives Through Redecision Therapy*, New York: Grove Press.
9. C. Moiso (1985), *Ego States and Transference*, Transactional Analysis Journal, 15(3) pp. 194-201.
10. E. Polster, and M. Polster (1973), *Gestalt Therapy Integrated*, New York: Random House.
11. R. May (1969), *Love and Will*, London: Collins.

whether most influenced by Freud[12] or Klein or Bion, consider the transference relationship to be the most important, if not the only, defining characteristic of the approach.

Clarkson in his book, *The Psychotherapeutic Relationship*, puts forward a review of five kinds of psychotherapeutic relationships given below which may be potentially available for constructive use in psychotherapy. In his words, "It is my belief that these five modalities of relationships exist in every psychotherapeutic relationship (whether it be with individuals, groups, families or larger systems). Like the keys on a piano, some of them may be played more frequently or more loudly than others, depending on the nature of the music. But they are always potentially there in every therapeutic encounter whether or not the pianist uses them, whether or not the composer acknowledges their existence in the written score. In this way, I think, the variety and nature of psychotherapeutic relationship is present implicitly or explicitly throughout the psychotherapeutic canon."[13]

The five famous forms or modalities of psychotherapeutic relationship that Clarkson has put forward are:

i. The working alliance,

ii. The transferential/counter transferential relationship,

iii. The reparative/developmentally needed relationship,

iv. The I–You relationship, and

v. The transpersonal relationship.

---

12. S. Freud (1912a), "The Dynamics of Transference," pp. 97-108 in J. Strachey (ed.), *The Standard Edition of the Complete Psychological Work of Freud,* vol. 12, London: Hograth Press.

13. Clarkson Petruska, "*The Psychotherapeutic Relationship.*"

This listing out may not be a comprehensive one, but I am not going into the detail of that, only I would like to mention a little about "the working alliance" which is probably the most essential relationship modality in psychotherapy. Without such a working alliance, psychotherapy is certainly limited in its goal and restricted in scope. This working alliance is represented by the client's or patient's willingness to engage in the psychotherapeutic relationship even when they at some archaic level may no longer wish to do so.

The working alliance may be conceptualized as a contract or agreement between the psychotherapist and the client. Now such willingness of the client or agreement or bond between the therapist and the client cannot be established and maintained, if confidentiality is not maintained from the therapist's end. If patients do not believe that therapists would keep their secrets then they would not divulge embarrassing but potentially medically important information, thus reducing their chances of getting the best medical care. So, confidentiality is an essential factor for psychotherapeutic relationship which is again crucial for the success of effective therapy. Thus we can say,

> Therapy presupposes relationship (Therapist-Client).
> Ralationship (Therapist-Client) presupposes confidentiality.
> Therefore, therapy presupposes confidentiality.

Hence, we can understand that the role of confidentiality is very crucial in Therapist-Client relationship. In the next section, we are going to clarify what confidentiality is.

Confidentiality

"Confidentiality" is the ethical reponsibility of psychotherapists to safeguard information they receive in the course of their practice (including teaching and research, as well as therapy).

Confidentiality, which is central to developing a trusting and productive Client-Therapist relationship is both a legal and an ethical issue. State laws now address confidentiality in therapy, as do the ethical codes of all the mental health professions.

Because no genuine therapy can occur unless clients trust in the privacy of their revelations to their therapists, professionals have the responsibility to define the degree of confidentiality that can be promised. Psychotherapists have an ethical responsibility to discuss the nature and purpose of confidentiality with their clients early in the counselling process. In addition, clients have a right to know whether their therapist may be discussing certain details of the relationship with supervisors or a colleague. Both the American Psychiatrist's Association (APA) and the American Counsellor's Association (ACA) have codes relevant to this subject. The APA's (1992) principle is: "Unless it is not possible or is contradicted, the discussion of confidentiality occurs at the outset of the relationship and thereafter as new circumstances may warrant."[14] The ACA's (1995) ethical code states: "When counselling is initiated and throughout the counselling process, it is necessary that the counsellors inform clients of the limitations of confidentiality and identify foreseeable situations in which confidentiality must be breached."[15]

In layman's term and client's interpretation — keeping confidence means "telling no one." "Confidentiality" is defined in the Oxford English Dictionary as: "Spoken or given in confidence, private, entrusted with secrets, confiding."[16] Another definition found in a social dictionary is that

14. *American Psychiatrist's Association.*

15. *American Counsellor's Association.*

16. *Oxford English Dictionary.*

"Confidentiality is the safeguarding of privacy in relation to information about service users."[17] (Thomas and Pierson, 1995, p. 87). Referring to the concept of "confidentiality," *International Encyclopaedia of Ethics* declares that the state or quality of communication being secret; the expectations that disclosure in the certain relationships will remain private.[18]

Now, what is "privacy?" The general notion of "privacy" refers to the state of being separate from the physical company or observation of others; more specifically, it refers to freedom from unauthorised intrusion.[19] Privacy alludes to personal investments that must not be intruded on by others. The right to privacy is a most cherished tradition with many laws protecting a person's privacy.

However, privacy can be breached under certain legal situations. For example, when a crime is about to be committed, the individual may relinquish the right to privacy. The very act of coming to a psychotherapist for treatment involves the surrender by the patient of his or her privacy. But in doing so, the patient expects a strict obligation on the part of the therapist that no communication or information imparted by the patient to the therapist may be shared with any outside individual or agency. This obligation not to reveal is what is meant by confidentiality, and, in the words of the Hippocratic oath, all these communications are "to be as holy secrets."[20] The patient has a compelling need to come to the therapist and speak freely because of emotional distress.

---

17. *Social Dictionary*, ed., by Thomas and Pierson, p. 87, 1995.
18. *International Encyclopaedia of Ethics*, ed., by J.K. Roth, Fitzroy Dearborn Publishers, p. 180, 1995.
19. *Webster's Dictionary*, 1989.
20. Hippocrates, *Corpus Hippocratinum*, 400 BCE.

However, the information communicated does not belong to the therapist, and in a number of legal situations this confidential exchange is protected from all demands, including those of the courts. Thus, this communication is then considered privileged. This privilege of not revealing information is what is referred to by such terms as physician-patient privilege, psychotherapist-patient privilege, priest-patient privilege, and attorney-client privilege.

Now, what do we understand by the term "privilege?" Is there any relationship between confidentiality and privilege? These two related stipulations are designed to safeguard information shared with the psychotherapist: "confidentiality and privilege." Confidentiality is concerned with the protection of patient's disclosure in a therapeutic setting, and privilege extends that protection to decisions about specific material to be potentially released, usually for judicial or quasi-judicial purposes. Confidentiality has a long ethical history in the medical field, while privilege is of relatively recent legal origin.

So, coming back to our original discussion related to confidentiality is that of "privacy" and "secrecy's" more paranoid conceptualization. Lined up against such concepts is the principle of openness — within society and its institutions.

The issue of openness versus privacy should always be topical in any democracy. This is an attempt to address a particular aspect of this wider scene — that of confidentiality within the mental health system. Lord Bingham, a lawyer, puts forward the limits of openness: "So similar is this principle of openness to those of us brought up in the common law that we sometimes forget how contrary is it to the principles on which the rest of our lines are conducted. It is very hard to think of any professional relationship which does not have a duty of confidence as one of its ingredients, probably a legal duty, but certainly an ethical duty. Doctors, lawyers, accountants, bankers, social workers, probationary officers, spiritual counsellors, officers of government, etc. would all recognize a clear obligation to preserve the confidentiality of matters imparted to them in confidence. And to some extent we respect the same rules in our private lives, looking askance at those who betray the confidence of their friends and acquaintances, even when they do not earn money by doing so. We do not, most of us, run our lives on a basis of total disclosure."[21]

Thus, from the above reflection it can be contended that in psychotherapy askance for confidentiality is not a very high demand. It is actually rooted in human nature. Trying to protect the respect of confidentiality is a common and ordinary social attitude of people. Thus, demand for confidentiality is not a very strict and stringent kind of demand, the price of which is not that high. So, we can say that in psychotherapy, when the therapist guarantees us the client's/patient's confidentiality, then we feel very safe and comfortable. But although we may observe that askance for confidentiality is rooted in human nature, it is not acceptable that confidentiality in psychotherapy is same as confidentiality in other professions, and that confidentiality in psychotherapy is not unique in nature.

As it has been mentioned earlier, here once more it should be spelt out very clearly that "confidentiality in psychotherapy" is clearly distinct from confidentiality in other professions.

In this context, we may refer to Julian Stern. Stern, in his book *Themes of Confidentiality in Clinical Practice* introduces the

---

21. Lord Bingham of Cornhill, (1996) "*Confidentiality" — An Inter-disciplinary Issue*?" The Inaugural Spring Lecture, Family Law, 315. National Council for Family Proceedings, pp. 2-8.

concept of absolute and relative confidentiality.[22] Following his view, it can be retorted that confidentiality in psychotherapy is relative in nature. While confidentiality in fields like law practice is absolute in nature, the lawyers have absolute respect for client's right to confidentiality. This can be contrasted with legal and moral positions of practising therapists. Psychotherapists, according to Stern, are much less clear about an absolute position. It is really difficult for them to maintain a clear-cut, absolute position because of the nature of the issues involved in the profession of psychotherapy. The position of lawyers, especially of criminal lawyers seems to be free of conflict of loyalty or interests.

If in psychotherapy, relative confidentiality is to be accepted, the role of confidentiality does not become less significant. In the process of discussing the significance of "confidentiality," we can say that a person (usually the client in a professional relationship) reveals sensitive information only because of trust that the disclosed information will remain private. Many professions today have ethical rules requiring their members not to disclose confidential communications roughly the same thing as keeping a secret under most circumstances. Like "privacy," here another term is being introduced. It is "secrecy" which has a close affinity with "confidentiality," but actually is different from it. In fact, "secrecy" and "privacy" are both certain features of "confidentiality." According to the *International Encyclopaedia of Ethics*, "A secret is information that is told to someone else with the reasonable expectancy that it will be private."[23] Again,

22. J. Stern, *Themes of Confidentiality in Clinicu. Practice.*

23. *International Encyclopaedia of Ethics*, ed. by J.K. Roth, Fitzroy Dearborn Publishers, 1995.

"privacy" as mentioned earlier refers to freedom from unauthorized intrusion.

On "secrecy," a law Lord has quoted Jeremy Bentham: "In the darkness of secrecy, sinister interest and evil in every shape have full swing. Only in proportion as publicity has a place can any of the checks applicable to judicial justice operate. Where there is no publicity, there is no justice . . . publicity is the very soul of justice. It is the keenest space to exertion and the surest of all grounds against improbity. It keeps the judge himself while trying under-trial."[24] (Shaw 1913). Again, anything disclosed, when other people overhear, it is not confidential.

Now, a confidential information is both private and secret. But what is more about confidentiality? The concept of "confidentiality" is strictly concealed with professional ethics. It is only relevant in the professional world. Secrecy and privacy are also both relevant in the realm of professional ethics but they are not restricted or confined to that only. They are also relevant in the public domain of normal day-to-day life situation. In normal communication, interaction, conversation, "privacy" and "secrecy" have significant contribution. These are the contexts like — priestly confession, sharing a secret with a friend. Thus, a demarcation should be made between "confidentiality" on the one hand, and "secrecy" and "privacy" on the other.

Moreover this difference can also be drawn on the basis of need-structure. This point can be clarified looking at the "need-structure" of the three concepts, viz. "confidentiality," "privacy" and "secrecy."

---

24. Shaw, Lord of Dunfermline, (1913), *Scott. vs. Scott.* (1913), AC 477.

In a case of confidentiality, need is there from both sides — client's side and the therapist's side.

1. ***From Client's Side***: From client's side there is a need that the information that he or she is exposing should be kept confidential. This need is founded on some definite ground, that the client is in a genuine need to be helped by the therapist. If the therapist fails to develop the therapist-client bond or relationship by maintaining some basic professional codes like keeping confidence, then the client's purpose of getting help from the therapist would not be fulfilled. Accordingly, some other purpose like — to have better mental health by getting rid from acute pain and suffering, cannot be attained. Thus, confidentiality is a very strong need from the client's side.

2. ***From Therapist's Side***: It is no wonder from common sensical view that the patient always wants to protect himself by expecting that the therapist should keep confidentiality. But at the same time, it is very significant that the therapist too would like to keep confidentiality. So, there is a need for keeping confidentiality from the therapist's side even. Such need is two-folded.

   a) There is a need for the therapist, to get as much confidential information as possible from the client for the purpose of therapy. This becomes possible by forming a proper client-therapist bond, the keyword for which is trust and empathy. Again this trust will be there if the therapist keeps confidentiality besides conforming to certain other professional codes. Thus, it seems that in the first place such need of the therapist is professional. If the client cannot entrust himself to the therapist professionally, then the latter would not be able to extract the information that is important for the purpose of his therapy. Consequently, the therapist would fail to make any progress in the course of his therapy. Thus technically speaking, confidentiality is a professional need for the therapist.

b) In the second place, not only getting confidential information but also maintaining it properly is important too. This need is related to achieving the therapeutic goal. Initially to start with and also for advancing in therapy, getting confidential information is important. But after that it is the therapist's major responsibility to maintain the confidentiality of such information with great sincerity. If the therapist will not succeed in maintaining confidentiality, then the client may discontinue his sessions due to lack of trust. He may face emotional set-back and accordingly have worse mental health, experiencing such mistrust. In any case, the therapist at any length cannot achieve the therapeutic goal. Thus, maintaining confidentiality is a need from the side of the therapist for the purpose of attaining therapeutic goal.

So, it can be said that in case of confidentiality, need is there from both the client's and the therapist's sides.

But in case of "privacy-secrecy," the need is only one-sided. It is only from the side of that person who is sharing the information, and not from the person who is receiving it. The person, who is sharing, has need or urge that the information shared is to be kept secret; they are something private. If privacy or secrecy is not maintained, the person concerned may face trouble. While the person to whom the information is given, does not feel any such need or urge for himself, this person will not be a gainer in any sense, if he keeps it private or secret. He will not even be a loser if he does not do so other than affecting or sacrificing the relationship itself. That person may maintain it in good faith only for the sake of the other one who actually shared the secret information. Here, we have to keep in mind that generally speaking, most of these cases are not professional. Such relationships are only of an informal nature. This person may maintain it, considering it as a mere principle of trust, in a loose sense, based on which general or normal human relationship is formed. Thus, "need" in case of "privacy-secrecy" is only one-sided.

In this way, from the point of view of "need-structure," the difference between "confidentiality" on the one hand and "privacy-secrecy" on the other can be seen.

Thus, we can understand that a pre-requisite for successful therapy is total confidence in revealing the most intimate, embarrassing, humiliating experiences, thoughts, dreams and fantasies. If the patient has any doubt or fears that anyone else could learn anything about the communication with the psychiatrist, it will have a chilling effect on the therapy, and may well prove an insurmountable obstacle to a successful outcome. Concern is not limited only to the possibility of embarrassment, humiliation or harm to the patient but also extends to the other individuals. Since the patient exposes not only his or her own private life but also reveals the secrets and intimate lives of others with whom he/she is involved.

So in this way confidentiality constitutes a patient's expectations and rights, its protection a professional duty on the part of the psychiatrist, and its violation an ethical transgression.

Confidentiality, Informed Consent and Truth-Telling

Now we see that the principle of medical confidentiality, that therapists must keep their client's secret, is one of the most venerable moral obligations of medical ethics. The obligation seems to be widely regarded as being exceedingly strict. According to the World Medical Association's *International Code of Medical Ethics*, it is an absolute requirement even after the patient's death. But though medical confidentiality is an important medico-moral principle that can be justified by its contribution to improving the patient's process of healing and respecting his/her autonomy and privacy, it may not be an absolute obligation. The General Medical Council's (GMC's) blue book lists the following eight exceptions to confidentiality.[25] These are:

a. When the patient or "his legal adviser" gives written and valid consent,

b. When other doctors or other health care professionals are participating in the patient's care,

c. When the doctor believes that a close relative or friend should know about the patient's health but it is medically undesirable to seek the patient's consent,

d. Exceptionally when the doctor believes that disclosure to a third party other than a relative would be in the "best interest of the patient" and when the patient has rejected "every reasonable effort to persuade,"

25. *General Medical Council.*

e. When there are statutory requirements to disclose information,

f. When a judge or equivalent legal authority directs a doctor to disclose confidential medical information,

g. (Rarely) when the public interest overrides the duty of confidentiality such as "investigation by the police of a grave or very serious crime," and

h. For the purposes of medical research approved by a recognized ethical committee.

In the mental health context we may say that it is almost a unanimous view. But broadly speaking, in case of (a) harm to public peril, and (b) harm towards private peril, the confidential information can be divulged by the therapist. Here the question may arise as to whether it should be ethical from the therapist's end to waive client's confidentiality when it goes against public good? Whether the individual (here the client) should get the priority or the society? Is it only specific beneficence that the therapist keeps in mind or general beneficence too? Now, here these questions and many other problems may occur. Important moral dilemmas may branch out as to whether such "breach of confidentiality" (whether in private or in public peril) is moral or immoral from the therapist's end. Solution to such problems is really very difficult and complicated. But, presently I am not concerned with those factors. Here, I would like to focus on a different issue. Taking into consideration the fact that divulging of confidential information may take place, I would like to analyse some situations in psychotherapeutic context where philosophical debate may break out centering around some important moral values like "truth and trust."

Now, divulgence of confidential information from the therapist's end may take place either: (a) with the informed consent of the client, or (b) without the consent of the client. If "breach of confidentiality" takes place with the consent of the client, then there would be no problem from either side. Because that is the ideal situation which is very much wanted in therapeutic context.

But problem occurs when "breach of confidentiality" takes place without the client's consent. In the mental health context, this happens in case of incompetent clients, i.e. those who are not in a position to give informed consent. It is generally believed that minors and psychotic clients are not in a position to give informed consent. Even competent clients may not consent to divulge confidentiality to any third party (carer like the parents). Like — (a) A teenaged boy, who disclosed information to his therapist about his recent dependence on drug, may not consent to pass on this information to anybody else; (b) A teenaged girl may not give consent for her therapist to divulge the information about her past history of taking oral contraceptive pills; (c) An adult may not wish that the information about his/her attempt of suicide that he/she disclosed to his/her therapist might be divulged in anyway. In such cases, the therapist may have a strong feeling that such information should be passed on to an authentic third party; here confidentiality should be waived in the course of treatment or therapy.

In such cases when confidentiality is waived without consent, a different issue emerges which has deep philosophical significance. Here we may observe two situations:

In one case, the client may come to know later that information is divulged without his consent. This situation may be seen in case of the teenaged boy just mentioned. In such a case, the relationship between therapist and client may be harmed as the client may have a feeling of betrayal by his therapist. The therapist may not remain trustworthy for the client anymore. The client may feel that he was being deceived as the therapist broke his promise (explicit or implict) regarding keeping his information confidential.

Another situation may be observed in this context, which may not be that complicated from the practical aspect, but from the moral point of view, it is as serious as the earlier one. This situation we may find in the third case mentioned earlier. The client may not wish to let his therapist divulge the information about his suicide attempts to any other person. But the therapist may feel the requirement and pass on the information to a carer of the client in the course of therapy. But at the same time the therapist may conceal or suppress this fact from his client and may continue the therapy in a proper direction. Here the client is having the idea that his therapist is keeping his explicit promise regarding confidentiality, but in reality this idea has been contradicted by the therapist's activity of which he is not aware. Does the therapist face any moral dilemma as being untruthful to his client when he has a stance on pretension, perhaps during other therapy sessions?

So, in these two situations cited above, we may find some ethical problems regarding truth telling in the context of confidentiality in therapist-client relation. Analysing the above cases, we may put three pointed questions in this context. These are:

1. Is the deliberate concealment of truth necessarily dishonest?
2. Is lying for the benefit of the patient a betrayal of trust?

3. How should therapists resolve conflict between their duty to be truthful and their other duties?

In response to the above-mentioned problems, it can be said that in all the situations the therapist's activity may be considered as moral if he engages himself for the client's beneficence. If client's beneficence remains the main aim of the therapist, then we can say that lying, promise breaking or breach of trust actually does not occur, though it may apparently seem to have occurred. In bio-ethics, the focus is usually upon general norms and values. Principle, for example, tries to develop methods to make norms and values explicit, and to weigh them in the concrete situations. Following this line of thought we may opine that truth is an important value, but it can be overruled by other values, especially that of "acting in the patient's best interest." If situation demands the therapist may choose to follow the principle of beneficence, which means that he/she acts in the patient's best interest, and by doing this the therapist is not disrespecting his/her patient's autonomy, which means that patient is regarded as a client whose wishes are to be respected by the therapist. But by this it does not mean the therapist has to keep each and every wish of the client in each occasion, especially those which are going against his/her process of healing. So if "cure/healing" is to be considered as the ultimate goal of successful therapy, then looking at "client's best interest" for his/her "health care need," we can conclude that the therapist in these cases, cannot be considered as a deceiver or untrustful. Here looking at a greater purpose, i. e. "client beneficence," we can say that —

a. Deliberate concealment of truth is not necessarily dishonesty, and

b. Lying (in the sense of suppression of truth) for the benefit of the patient is not a betrayal of trust.

Therefore, in order to resolve the conflict of the therapist between his duty to be truthful and his other duties, it can be said that it is "health care need" of the client, which should be given maximum preference than any other factor. From the theoretical perspective, it should be valued most and also from the practical perspective of a practitioner or professional too. Thus, a clinical ethicist can suggest or prescribe that in case of such a significant issue of medical ethics like confidentiality-related problem cited above in therapist-client relationship, "patient's best interest" has to be served by the therapist. Lastly, it should be mentioned here that in this paper, I have not gone into the detailed account of the conceptual differences, made by the moralists, between being truthful and not to lie, and also between lying, deceiving, concealing, pretending, etc. A lot of analyses can be made in this regard. Here, actually I have tried to philosophically conceptualize some practical problems that may emerge in physician-patient relationship in mental health context and also tried to bring out certain insights from the ethical point of view, which can be considered as a contribution in the field of applied ethics or applied philosophy.

10

Glimpse into the Domain of Consent in the Doctor-Patient Relationship
Is it a Myth or a Reality?

Nandini Banerjee

THE issue of consent has attracted a lot of discussion in medical circles, the media and the general public in recent times. Though the concept has been known to exist in the times of Hippocratic medicines, the scope and principles governing practice expanded in recent times to keep pace with the rapid scientific and technological advancements in medicine in the last fifty years. With the growth of medical ethics in the 1960's consent has come to play a pivotal role in clinical practice.

The history of the doctor-patient communication dates back to antiquity. It has been an age-old practice for doctors to make decisions for their patients and it is deeply embedded in the Hippocratic oath — *I swear by Apollo and Asclepius that I will follow that system of regimen which according to my ability and judgement I consider for the benefit of my patients,* and this view was endorsed several centuries later in 1847 by the American Medical Association. The unbridgeable gap between the doctor and the patient thus remained unchanged with active support from the profession.

The recognition of human beings as autonomous agents capable of self-determination is a notion of the 20th century — it was engineered as a desirable quality to have, rather than deserving respect, until recently. As late as the 1950's social scientists like Parsons opined that *A physician is a technically competent person whose competence and specific judgements cannot be competently judged by the layman and therefore should take such judgements as authority.* Dostyovesky claims illness as one of the most fearful moments of life needing "mystery, miracle and authority."[1] Such an attitude in the current arena of ethics would be considered more of a hindrance than a facilitator in doctor-patient communication.

Medical Science in itself has grown over the years with diagnosis of new diseases and disease-causing organisms; advanced modalities of treatment resulting in a possible cure in many a hitherto incurable malady and the changing perception of disease in the community at large. A more objective assessment is possible at the bedside nowadays, to predict the likely outcome of cure or to anticipate whether a treatment is futile or impossible. In spite of such changes being made, medicine continued to remain enmeshed in the world of numeric, charts and algorithms, ignoring the fact that it still needed as in the days of Hippocrates, subjective data from patients to base subjective judgements.

The winds of change were brought in from the legal fraternity when the rulings in two successive cases in the USA attempted to define the boundaries of informed consent in clinical practice. This was a landmark judgement, which advised doctors to disclose and explain to the patient in a language as

---

1. B. Steinbock, J.D. Arras and A.J. London, *Ethical Issues in Modern Medicine*, 6th ed., Mc Graw Hill, pp. 93-94.

simple as necessary, the nature of the ailment, the nature of the proposed treatment, the probabilities of success or failure and alternatives if available. These cases in 1957 and 1960 in California and Kansas had failed to disclose the risks inherent with the proposed treatment and had resulted in harmful consequences for the patient. Professional guidelines were laid in conjunction with common law to enable clinicians to take appropriate decisions when dealing with individual patients. The role of playing God on earth was transformed to share decision-making based on mutual trust and respect. More recently, the growth of patients rights movements, an increasing consumerist attitude towards medicine and abuses and controversial cases like those of Alder Hey and Bristol in the UK, have thrown up a lot of debate on the issue of consent and emphasise the need to reassess and review the current practice.

The next section discusses the ethical principles governing consent and the professional guidelines and law in this regard.

Ethical Framework of Consent

The edifice of modern medicine is based on four ethical pillars namely autonomy, beneficence, non-maleficence and justice. Consent respects autonomy and ensures non-maleficence. The focus on autonomy reflects deontological reasoning and makes consent absolutely necessary (to treat individuals as ends in themselves) while focussing on non-maleficence reflects consequential reasoning, making consent, relatively valuable (individual benefit is judged in relation to societal benefit/ conflict of individual gain *versus* societal harm). Its importance lies in the fact that it ensures decisions to be taken in a consistent manner and guards against occasions when one might be tempted not to take consent.[2] It needs to be remembered however that peoples' cultural environments substantially influence their autonomous beliefs, including their moral stances. In recognising and respecting autonomy, the frail human nature ensures a *prima facie* moral requirement to respect both individual and cultural moral variability.[3]

Legal Aspects of Consent

Consent respects autonomy. However autonomy has never been fully recognized as a legally protectable entity. The law has rules to subserve bodily integrity and prevent bodily harm. The legal position is not enshrined in statute, but emerges from common law based on professional duty of care, breach of that duty without malice or intent to cause harm but results in preventable or foreseeable harm resulting in loss of bodily integrity or death.

The issue of consent is dealt with both in Civil and Criminal Law — charges of battery and assault (non consensual touching, consent under fear or duress or incompetent to give consent, procedure performed in spite of express refusal of consent, where patient was inadequately informed to provide an effective consent and where the clinician mistakes the scope of his/her authority) in civil cases are liable to pay damages or compensation whereas charges of negligence, manslaughter and murder in criminal law are punishable by imprisonment. There is a scope for raising issues of consent in the context of

---

2. *Handbook of Dilemmas in Health Care Ethics,* University of Birmingham, UK, Consent: Ethics and Law, 2005: pp. 11-12.
3. R. Gillion, "Ethics Needs Principles — Four can encompass the Rest — And Respect for Autonomy Should be First Among Equals." *J. Med Ethics,* 2003, 29: pp. 307-12.

Article 2 (Right to Life), Article 3 (Prohibition of Torture and Inhuman or Degrading Treatment) and Article 10 (Right to Freedom of Expression) of The Human Rights Act, 1998. There has been no case law as yet and none of the texts have identified consent to medical treatment as a target for litigation.[4]

The following guidelines are legally binding on the health care professionals practising in the United Kingdom:[5]

- Consent is a mandatory requirement before examining and treating competent adults.
- Adults are assumed to be competent unless demonstrated otherwise.
- Patients incompetent in other matters of personal or family life may be competent in health care matters.
- Consent is a process, not a one off event; efforts must be made to ensure validity of consent.
- Children aged 16 and 17 are capable of giving consent. Younger children can give consent if presumed competent. Parents can override this decision. However, parents cannot override consent to refusal of treatment.
- It is right for the clinician treating the patient or performing the procedure to seek consent.
- Adequate information is to be provided to make a reasonable choice.
- Consent must be obtained voluntarily.

---

4. *Handbook of Dilemmas in Health Care Ethics*, University of Birmingham, UK, Consent: Ethics and Law, 2005: p. 15.
5. *Good practice in Consent Implementation Guide*, Appendix A, 12 "Key Points on Consent: the Law in England."

- Consent can be written, oral or non-verbal.
- Competent adults including pregnant women have the right to refuse treatment despite obvious benefits.
- No one can give consent on behalf of an incompetent adult; their best interests guide their treatment.
- Advance refusal by incompetent patients when they were competent is binding on the clinician if it refers to the situation under consideration.
- Consent regarding use of human tissue or organs is governed by agreement or refusal of patients or their next of kin to use such material for education and research. If consent is given, such samples should be anonymised.
- Written consent is needed for photographic or video recording of a patient for education, publication or research purposes. Patients may wish to see such material and stop their use at any point even after initial consent.

Role of Professional Bodies

Realising the fact that consent would soon become the centre stage of the doctor-patient relationship, it became imperative on the medical profession to devise guidelines to ensure that consent was effectively practised.

The British Medical Association (BMA) has done some leading work in this area and emphasises the fact that consent is not merely signing a document but a complete understanding of the ins and outs of the proposed care. Clinicians, according to the BMA, need to have a thorough insight into legal and ethical implications in this context and should refrain from delegating responsibility to junior colleagues who lack experience in such matters. Apart from the legal requirements of the consenting process, every opportunity must be provided to the patient by the care-giver to ask questions and a great deal of care taken to provide the initial information in a comprehensive manner. Not only the doctor involved in direct care of the patient is responsible, but also other members of the team should be knowledgeable to expand on the information provided and clear the doubts.

The General Medical Council (GMC) states that successful relationships between doctors and patients are based on trust. In order to establish the trust, patient's rights to make an informed choice should be respected and the GMC outlines the legal standard of requirement as the minimum standard for good practice. Open helpful dialogue with patients leads to clarity of objectives and greater understanding, strengthening the doctor-patient relationship by providing an agreed framework of action. Patients are likely to adhere to treatment plans if they have been taken into confidence. The key to consent as depicted in the GMC's good practice guidelines lies in providing sufficient information, prioritising patient needs based on individual beliefs, culture, occupation and other factors that have a bearing on his/her daily life. Withholding information is justifiable in the context of harmful consequences or deteriorating health resulting from disclosure of such information. It considers obtaining consent voluntarily as absolutely necessary and agrees to provide medical treatment without consent only as a life-saving or stabilising measure in an emergency. Regarding incompetent adults and in organ procurement for education and research, it echoes the same views as expressed in the BMA document.[6]

---

6. "Seeking Patients Consent": The Ethical Considerations, *General Medical Council Guidance to Doctors*, GMC Publications, UK.

Why is Consent Important?

The standard argument favouring consent is respecting patient autonomy; however, it is a model contract that has enshrined in it legitimate expectations — conflicting, harmonious or otherwise that would empower patients to play an active part in decision-making. It is a well known fact that in the clinical setting of injury or illness there is an accompanying loss of status and a diminished sense of personhood more so in patients already marginalized on account of race, class and/or gender. The purpose of consent then is to assure the patient reasonably that he has not been deceived or coerced into accepting something that was not his intent. If empowerment is viewed as justice then restoring the patient's control over his/her self by maximal participation in the decision-making process is the way forward to deliver justice. This has wider implications in access to health care and institutional structures beyond the individual doctor-patient encounter.[7]

The concept of informed consent can also be looked upon as the expression of the professional virtue of fidelity; being a covenant it denotes the solemn and binding agreement between individuals. Such a relationship according to some authors is not merely transactional as it considers deeper needs outside the self-perceived needs of the patient.

Last but not the least, the ethic of care is demonstrated in consent in the relationship under discussion.

---

7. K. Labacqz, "Empowerment in the Clinical Setting. Theology, Ethics and the Clinical Encounter," G.P. McKenny, J.R. Sande, ed., Theological Analysis of the Clinical Encounter, Dordrecht, Kluwer Academic Publishers, 1994: pp. 133-47.

Elements of Informed Consent

In this section, I would like to present the various types of consents in practice before discussing on the principal elements necessary to make consent valid in health care. There are important distinctions between express, tacit, implicit and presumed consent.

Express consent is the one commonly used — this utilizes the signature to express solidarity to the decision taken. *Tacit* consent is agreeing not to dissent from a proposed course of action and *implied* consent is expressed apparent compliance for investigation or treatment. *Presumed* consent is an assumption about a decision a person would make if he/she were capable of consenting.[8]

There are three principal elements in consent: notably, capacity or competence of the patient, doctor's ability to impart sufficient information to make an informed decision, and the decision thus adopted is truly voluntary — effective communication links them together.

Capacity or competence is of primary importance and perhaps the most controversial. This is because of the lack of objective measures to assess competence and poor reproducibility due to significant inter and intrapersonal variations in interpretation. Competence in itself is task-specific and changes over time. Patients are assumed to understand the information provided, retain them for an adequate length of time to arrive at an informed decision and to be able to appreciate the significance of the action chosen. The chosen action must be independent of any direct or indirect influences on the decision including coercion and/or incentives from

8. N.G. Messer, "Professional-patient Relationship and Informed Consent," *Postgraduate Medical Journal*, 2004, 80: pp. 277-83.

family, friends or the clinician. Coercion may range from innocuous persuasion by the physician by virtue of his knowledge and experience to gross exploitation by offering monetary benefits in organ donation and research, more likely to influence vulnerable sections of society.

At the other end of the paradigm, the professional should provide adequate relevant information in a simple manner and communicate it effectively. Opinions vary between clinicians regarding what is sufficient or adequate information for disclosure as there is a fear of too much or too tittle being provided. The minimum standard required is based on the "reasonable doctor" (Bolam principle) and the "prudent patient" model extended to include the "reasonable patient" and the "subjective standard" (what a particular person considers adequate). A word of caution needs to be sounded regarding the "reasonable person" — whereas some patients may consider disclosure of every detail acceptable, others may leave everything for the clinician to decide.

The secret of success in practice of consent lies in communicating this information tailored to the needs of the individual patient recognizing the limitations in each situation. The standards outlined are only guidelines for wise men to follow and fools to act upon. Communication should be honest, sympathetic, lucid, avoiding jargon of the medical lexicon, done consciously with time and effort in a comfortable environment. Evidence suggests that effective transfer of information depends on the amount of information provided at a given point of time, the intonation pattern and the sex of the professional imparting the information — women tending to do better. The aim is to make it as patient-centred as possible, rehearsing the facts with mutual respect, conveying a sense of equipoise, and transparency in the preservation of autonomy.

Problems with Consent in Clinical Practice

The domain of consent would remain incomplete without knowledge of the problems likely to be encountered in practice and the fundamental weaknesses inherent in the concept, and in this section I intend to provide these issues in a nutshell.

PROBLEMS IN THE CONCEPT

The insurmountable obstacle in the concept of consent is the inability to realize the scientific truth to the fullest extent. Medical Science is still profoundly ignorant of Nature and a lot of our understanding is in fact pretence or useless jargon to fill in the gaps of knowledge. The uncertainties in medical diagnostic effects of many a therapeutic procedure is a major hindrance to disclosure and consent. Sharing uncertainties needs a willingness to admit and convey, at the same time taking care not to overwhelm the recipient with more shades of grey than is needed to establish the reality. Implementation of the concept then becomes difficult with physicians caught between the dilemma of acknowledging uncertainty and at the same time struggling to maintain authority without compromising their effectiveness as healers.[9]

Even if it is desirable on balance to embark on the optimal pathway of shared decision-making, it cannot be ignored that illness and disease in itself results in loss of bodily harmony which in turn results in some loss of autonomy of the patient and/or family, making it obligatory for the medical profession to err on the side of beneficence or in least non-maleficence. It thus ensures paternalism to fulfil a need created by illness making the concept fatally compromised to start with.

---

9. B. Steinbock, J.D. Arras and A.J. London, *Ethical Issues in Modern Medicine*, 6th ed., Mc Graw Hill, pp. 96-97.

The concepts of Autonomy and Beneficence in the ethical context are self-contradictory — while autonomy would mean exercising personal liberties without limitations imposed by others, it may become necessary for beneficence to actually refrain people from exercising such liberties. Harm is not specified in *primum non nocere* of Hippocratic medicine and so also the intending benefits — is it physical integrity or dignitary integrity that amounts to beneficence? Or is it linked to benefits with restoration of physical well-being? — the questions remain unanswered with the clinician left to decide what is more important between the two in a given context.

PROBLEMS IN IMPLEMENTATION

The British Medical Association (BMA) has voiced some concerns with the current practice of consent by health care professionals in the UK. It has been pointed out that too much importance is placed on signing the consent form, that only proves communication has taken place on the subject between patient and physician, but does not ensure validity. Patients need time to reflect on information provided which means that the entire process is a continuum in time and not a timed event — this may appear idealistic in a modern health care system hard-pressed for time and resource limitations embodying other priorities. The kind of communication envisaged requires personal interaction that may prove costly in the professional's time and energy, raising ethical and political debate about organization of health care delivery.[10]

The five years of training in medical school while aiming to design safe physicians filled in with enormous knowledge of the mechanics of the human body, unfortunately does not

---

10. N.G. Messer, "Professional-patient relationship and Informed Consent," *Postgraduate Medical Journal,* 2004, 80: pp. 277-83.

train one to apply the knowledge holistically and face up to the challenges posed in clinical practice of imparting the information gathered in the years of rigorous training. Transfer of information is crucial in the whole process, more so under the stress of illness, where information is likely to be forgotten, misunderstood and difficult to comprehend.

There is a further problem of opacity of consent, where consent to an action A, also logically entails action B and consequence C — the patient having consented to A, has actually not consented to either B or C, whereas the professional, to whom the link is quite obvious takes for granted that the patient has consented to the entire process (note in issues of organ donation).[11]

It is important to realize, that, in spite of all said and done in the patient-doctor relationship, the former is the more vulnerable member in the relationship, there being an imbalance in knowledge and power gained by years of training and experience favouring the latter and therefore a measure of dependency on him/her. Voluntariness in such a situation may not be entirely voluntary and rational. Persuasion by the clinician in good faith can amount to unconsciously putting gentle influence or pressure in arriving at a decision. The matter becomes even more complicated in areas of research and organ donation where a mistaken fear of compromised care exists in the mind of the patient if she/he fails to comply with the clinician, and, where incentives in cash or kind are involved, may be induced to accepting unjustified risks or burdens. Members of prisons, the military and in some institutions with powerful authority structures may be coerced to consent in lieu of waiver of penalties and sentences.[12]

---

11. Ibid.
12. Ibid.

Conclusion

IS CONSENTING A MYTH?

From the foregoing discussion, it is amply evident that a gulf exists between theory and practice of consent in competent adults. There being many undefined boundaries, application of this principle in incompetent individuals tends to acquire mythical proportions.

It takes no more than common sense to understand that the next of kin or nominated representative could make decisions for them in such situations as is acceptable in many societies till date, even with competent adults. Family members making surrogate decisions must take great care to ensure that the patients and not the decision-maker's needs are paramount in determining the decision. There can be cases where the individual's needs may not be disentangled from the needs of the family and professional help needs to be sought to sort out the issue.

Regarding criteria for surrogate decision-making, a hierarchy of advance directives, substituted judgement and best interests are accepted as guidelines. Advance directives are only applicable if they are specific for the current situation and do not reflect the change of identity of a person over the time. Substituted judgement relies on the decision-maker stepping into the patient's shoes based on knowledge of the patient and his/her aims and values. Evaluation of best interest is made on the basis of value judgement about another life if worth living and imagining how it would least restrict his/her future choices.

Proxy consent has its own boundaries. The decisions are valid if and only if the proposed course of action, on balance of risks and benefits favours the latter while entailing harm no more than that ordinarily encountered. In case of children, there might be some justification for psychological benefit (altruistic motivation in donating an organ to another sibling) or moral development (participating in research for benefit of others).

WHAT CAN BE DONE TO MAKE "CONSENT" A REALITY?

Before drawing a line on the subject, I propose to put forward a few suggestions directed to both partners in the relation to make consent more reproducible in practice and more workable than a mere theoretical exercise.

For Professionals

- It should be made sure that the proposed investigation/treatment is what the patient wants, solely not what he needs.
- Adequate information has been provided and understood — cross check/repeat the discussion if in doubt initially — go ahead when absolutely sure.
- Decide for yourself that the proposed modality is the best one of the many courses of action after referring to guidelines or evidence available on the subject — convey this to the patient.
- If non-treatment is the preferred option, explain why it is so compared to available treatment in the patient's context.
- Involve patient's family and take help from colleagues and legal advice where necessary.
- Be honest about knowledge or lack of it/limitations to expertise and discuss with seniors/colleagues if unsure.

- Educate and empower patients to opt out or take second opinions if they feel the need to do so — explain that this would not alter care plan.
- Establish dialogue with medical schools, national professional bodies to impart training and improve communication skills for doctors in training and organize mandatory assessment/regular appraisals as part of the medical curriculum.
- An audit on current practice to identify problems, highlight weaknesses and recommend changes.
- A comprehensive manual to be provided to all medical graduates in addition to the Hippocratic oath to serve as a ready reckoner.

For Patients

- Views should be voiced without fear of losing trust or faith in the relation.
- Every opportunity should be taken to express concerns and clarify doubts.
- Must be able to understand the scope of the proposed action and willing to negotiate.
- The clinician should be viewed not as superior or as an adversary but as a fellow human being with specialist skills and expertise.
- That life is not without morbidity, some of the treatments prolong death rather than sustain life and Nature takes its course when inevitable.

Albeit the relation between theory and practice is a complex one, becoming more contentious the deeper we dig in to retrieve the connections. Again and again we should remind ourselves that medicine is not an exact science, it lies in an area between science and art dealing with human life that has a body, mind and soul.

The public opinion is shaken now and then by the frequent bias of media reporting.[13] Consent could become a workable reality when patients participate in their care as well as in health planning and rationing while doctors give their best to make their encounters transparent. In its absence, consent would continue to remain in the words of Churchill *an enigma wrapped in mystery* while we waste our time chasing the moonshine.

13. Editorials: Working With and for Patients, *Clinical Medicine*, vol. 3, No. 6, Nov./Dec. 2003.

11

Patient-Physician Relationship for Conducting a Clinical Trial

A Look on Ethical Aspects and Role of Statistical Designs

Gopaldeb Chattopadhyay

THE circumstances surrounding the administration of experimental drug and treatment to human beings trouble the conscience of the different community of people, like theologians, sociologists, lawyers, economists, scientists and physicians. A patient wants to be cured when he approaches a physician. A physician wants to make the patient ailment-free. We must recognize that a physician takes care of patients. The patient who takes medicine has to believe that it has been given in good faith, that it is not poison meant to kill. Thus a patient-physician relationship builds up. They become partners in the social contracts, although strangers. The contract that makes medical care possible is the patient-physician relationship.

One of the important advances in medicine during the past decade has been the increased acceptance of the controlled clinical trials. Ethical issues are not nuisance imposed on research but are rules that guide interactions on human beings so as to say people experimenting on other people. Human interaction is complicated. Thus, we are not demanding anything which is new, but we are talking about something that makes clinical research fit the world for which it was designed; the world of people taking care of other people. Our intention is not to criticize the physician or the patient. We do not think what is done is bad. On the whole the system works surprisingly well except for a few atrocious cases. We just want to make sure that through our *collective applied cleverness* we somehow become able to devise alternatives that are arguably better for patients and scientifically responsible.

Section 2 of this article points out a few instances where unethical means have been taken to conduct clinical trial on human beings. The next section deals with the principles of bioethics. In section 4, we have discussed about physician's dilemma of treating a patient and a few additional ethical issues for conducting clinical trial. Section 5 is dedicated to the role of statistical methodologies for conducting clinical trial, while in section 6, we have discussed about some statistical techniques currently in use for conducting more ethical clinical trial. The article ends up with some concluding remarks.

II

Human Guinea Pigs in the History of Clinical Trial

In a clinical trial, when the subjects of interest are human beings, ethical issues get priority. On the whole, it is my belief that standard experimental practice takes reasonable care of the patients in clinical trials and what bothers is the conscience because it is not clear that the patient is receiving the best possible care in the experimental situation. However, there are a few atrocious cases that demand serious concern towards development of ethical patient-physician relationship.

The Tuskegee syphilis experiment — Brandt (1978), Jones, (1981): The study was conducted by U.S. Public Health Service (PHS) in 1932 and continued up to 1972, in Alabama, to determine the course and effects of untreated syphilis. The experiment stopped when the *Associated Press* broke the story. In the experiment, 400 black sharecroppers, most of whom were never informed that they had syphilis, were observed as the disease consumed them. In the 1950s when penicillin became widely recognized as the preferred treatment for syphilis, PHS actually prevented the test's participants from receiving the drug.

Throughout 1960s the University of Cincinnati conducted research for the Department of Defence in which largely indigent and terminally ill cancer patients were subjected to whole body radiation at near-lethal levels. There was no potential benefit to the participants, and the major purpose appears to have been to evaluate the effects of a nuclear attack — Ebersold (1973) and Kairys (1996).

History of similar experiments are abundant, often conducted on prisoners, including one in 1971 in which scurvy was induced in subjects so that researchers could observe its progress — Mitford (1974) and Kairys (1996).

In 1963, the Sloan-Kettering Institute for Cancer Research and the U.S. Public Health Service conducted a test to determine the human response to foreign cancerous cells; elderly and largely incompetent participants, who did not have cancer, were injected with cancerous cells, after researchers obtained oral consent by calling it a "skin test" and failing to disclose that cancerous cells would be injected — Kairys (1996).

A long list of highly unethical practices in experimentation on human subjects can be found in Beecher (1966) and Pappworth (1967). In response to widespread publicity about the Tuskegee study in 1972, U.S. Congress established the National Commission for the Protection of Human Subjects of Biomedical Research, which led to President's Commission for the Style of Ethical Problems in Medicine and Biomedical and Behavioral Research and to the adoption of new federal regulations in 1981.

So, the ethical issues in clinical trial, especially when the subjects are human beings are no longer a neglected issue, although it is accepted that for the progress of science experimentations cannot be stopped. In the next section we shall talk about bioethics.

III

Bioethics

There are two very general types of ethical theories. One based on evaluating the consequence of either individual acts or rules in the light of some very general goal such as happiness or pleasure. This "consequentialist" type has one influential subtype called "utilitarianism," in which, in the classical formulation of Mill, one should act to maximize the greatest happiness for the greatest number of people. Another quite different type of ethical theory is based on a very general set of rules that, it is argued, are right in themselves regardless of the consequences. This type of theory is called "deontological" and its pure form is associated historically with the name of Kant. At present, the Harvard philosopher John Rawls is associated with a deontological type of theory though Rawls' (1971) approach does not induce him to take consequences into account. Another form of deontologism that is quite influential in the area of biomedical ethics is due to Ross (1930), who developed a theory of prima-facie duties. Charles Fried in his (1974) book viewed the patient-physician relationship under the rubric of "personal care." "Personal Care" for Fried is construed as an individual right-based ethical relationship, i.e. "deontological" in nature. It is also elaborated in terms of some specific values, which he terms "rights." These "rights" are grouped under the following four rubrics:

i. ***Lucidity***: By this Fried meant "the right to know all relevant details about the situation which . . . (the patient) finds himself in." He sees this as a "constitutive" good: "to deny a patient the opportunity for lucidity is to treat him not as a person but as a means to an end."

ii. ***Autonomy***: This connotes freedom from force and violence.

iii. ***Fidelity***: This appears to be associated with notions of honesty, nondeceitfulness and trust, and is incompatible with lying.

iv. ***Humanity***: This refers to have a person's "full human particularity taken into account by those who enter into relationships with him." This notion of human particularity means the individualized "wants, needs, and vulnerabilities" associated with specific person.

A somewhat different, though overlapping, set of values was introduced by Beauchamp and Childress (1989) in connection with their more systematic treatment of biomedical ethics. Using something like Ross's system of prima-facie duties, these authors define four ethical principles that help us in making ethical decisions. These principles are:

i. ***Autonomy***: A person is autonomous if and only if he or she is self-governing. The individual then can legislate norms of conduct and is able to voluntarily fix a course of action.

ii. ***Non-maleficence***: This principle has Hippocratic basis and means "do no harm." This usually means both the prevention of harm and the removal of harmful conditions.

iii. ***Beneficence***: This refers to a duty to confer benefits or to help others further their important and legitimate interests.

iv. ***Justice***: This refers to giving each person his or her "right or due." One is just towards a person if one gives that person what the person deserves or is owed. This notion is further developed in a set "material principles of justice" such as " To each an equal share" or "To each according to merit."

Schaffner (1996) states,

> It would appear a rather general truth in biomedical ethics that high-level theories such as utilitarianism are too abstract to provide much guidance in resolving ethical conundra. At the same time, specific rules are too limited and constraining to be used as tools in ethical deliberations outside of rather circumscribed areas.

Dewey and Tufts (1936) make this point well in their characterization of the role of principles:

> Moral principles are the final methods used in judging suggested courses of action . . . Their object is to supply standpoints and methods, which will enable the individual to make for himself an analysis of the elements of good and evil in the particular situation in which he finds himself . . . No genuine moral principle prescribes a specific course of action; rules, like cooking recipes, may tell just what to do and how to do it. A moral principle such as that of chastity, of justice, of the Golden Rule [which is not a rule but a

> principle] gives the agent a basis for looking at and examining a particular question . . . It holds before him certain possible aspects of the act; it warns him against taking a short or partial view of the act. It economizes his thinking by supplying him with the main heads by reference to which to consider the bearings of his desires and purposes; it guides him in his thinking by suggesting to him the important considerations for which he should be on the lookout.
>
> A moral principle, then, is not a command to act or forbear acting in a given way; it is a tool for analyzing a special situation, the right or wrong being determined by the situation in its entirety, and not by the rule as such.

Levine and Lebacqz (1979) examined and analyzed a number of ethical problems with clinical trials with the aid of "four basic principles for human conduct: *doing good* (beneficence), *not harming* (non-maleficence), *respecting persons,* and *distributing goods and evils fairly* (justice)."

There is rough equivalence of Levine and Lebacqz's and Fried's concept with Beauchamp and Childress's approaches, despite some differences and this article is not meant for discussion of the same (interested reader can see Schaffner (1996). However, this suggests that we may well have at hand a reasonably robust methodology for dealing with the complex ethical issues in clinical trials.

IV

Physician's Dilemma

Sometimes the physician remains in dilemma due to his dual role of a healer and a scientist. As a healer, the physician is bound by various professional codes to act in the patient's best interest. The usual reference to support the claim is the

Hippocratic oath. Other codes such as the Declaration of Geneva of the World Medical Association and the International Code of Medical Ethics are quite clear that the physician must act in the best interest of the patient (see Katz, 1972).

As a scientist, the physician's main concern is to respect scientific canons of valid experimental design, which may require that the physician sacrifice the goal of individualized best treatment for statistical efficiency. Clayton (1982) in his essay characterizes these two different ethical responsibilities of the physician as follows:

i. ***Individual Ethics***: It is the duty of the doctor to apply existing knowledge for the best possible treatment of each individual patient.

ii. ***Collective Ethics***: (a) It is the duty of the doctor to acquire new knowledge so that, by such advance knowledge, future patients might benefit, and (b) having acquired new knowledge, to accurately communicate it to other doctors.

The two roles or "ethics" of the physician are not necessarily in harmony. In addition to keep a balance between the two roles of a physician, Schaffner in his (1996) article considered two additional general ethical issues: Beginning of a Trial, and Terminating a Trial.

The history of medicine is replete with clinical therapies that have won the uncritical acceptance of physicians. There was little systematic development of clinical investigation in 17$^{t\text{-}h}$ century. Francis Bacon (1623) proposed that more emphasis be placed on experience in the selection of treatments, and that learned physician's contribute information on remedies "tried and approved by experiment for the cure of particular diseases." And he cautioned: "This part therefore, which treats of authentic and positive medicines, I set down as wanting. But it is a thing that should not be undertaken without keen and severe judgement and in synod, as it were, of select physicians." Some in the eighteenth century recognized the need for controlled clinical experiments. A particularly interesting example is found in the writings of the British philosopher George Berkeley (1752), who was convinced of the great curing powers of tar-water. The modern scientific attitude towards medicine began emerging during the first decade of the 19th century in France, made possible to a large extent by the gradual development of a sound nosology. Examination of patients, classification of diseases and the observation of their natural course were assuming increased importance. This approach reached its culmination in the clinicopathologic investigations of P.C.A. Louis, who was the first to make extensive and systematic use of record keeping and data analysis, and to insist on their indispensability to medical methodology. The most famous application of Louis's (1836) method was to the practice of bleeding. He also developed guidelines to be followed in designing prospective studies for evaluating different modes of treatment (see Louis, 1834). Most recent examples include irradiation for infected tonsils in the 1940s, and the administration in the late 1940s and early 1950s of the synthetic estrogen diethylstilbestrol (DES) to prevent miscarriages. These therapies were not only ineffective but also have been linked to carcinoma in later years or (for DES) in the next generation. Courts have determined that tests on mice in 1939 had shown that DES crossed the placenta and "had malforming action on the foetus" and the drug companies marketing DES should have conducted additional experiments to test the safety of DES prior to marketing the substance (see Schaffner (1987) for a discussion of DES and references). Prevention of ineffective and potentially dangerous therapies is required, and clinical trials are conceded by virtually everyone to be the best procedure to achieve this end. The necessity for clinical trials is supported by several professional ethical codes. The Declaration of Helsinki, for example, states:

> Biomedical research involving human subjects must conform to generally accepted scientific principles and should be based on adequately performed laboratory and animal experimentation and on a thorough knowledge of the scientific literature.

Though these general principles are unquestionable, exactly when and under what circumstances a clinical trial should begin and what type of clinical trial it should be are intensely debated topics. Similarly, when to terminate a trial is also a valued question because if we can terminate the trial in proper time with a proper scientific conclusion then, early termination will help us to introduce the more effective treatment procedure and to drop the less effective treatment procedure at the earliest resulting in saving more lives. The third concern, i.e. the ethical difficulty of a physician to play the role of a healer and a scientist is also an important issue and the question comes whether it is possible to assign a treatment based on information generated by the trial to that point, so that ultimately we can treat lesser number of patients by the inferior treatment and also the scientific goal is achieved. Statistics can perhaps play some role in these issues.

V

Role of Statistics in Clinical Trial

Acquisition of new knowledge is the goal of any scientific activity. In empirical scientific research, new knowledge or scientific results are generated by an investigation or study. A clinical trial is basically an experiment designed to evaluate the beneficial and adverse effects of a new medical treatment or intervention. Generally clinical trials are categorized in four types, viz. Phase I, Phase II, Phase III and Phase IV trials. Phase I trials are exploratory and are concerned with aspects of clinical pharmacology and toxicity. Phase II studies are concerned with evaluating both efficacy and safety aspects. Phase III trial is the definitive evaluation of the proposed new therapy in which effectiveness is verified and presence of any long-term side effects is monitored. Patients suffering from the disease in question are randomly assigned either to the new experimental treatment or to the current standard treatment or possibly placebo. Occasionally, more than two treatments will be compared in the same study. It is in the comparative Phase III study that the statistical design and analysis have been paid due attention and scrutiny. Phase IV refers to the additional testing and monitoring of experience with the new treatment after it has been accepted and approved for general use, sometimes referred to as post-marketing surveillance. This categorization is not a strict one, and a trial's purpose can overlap the boundary definitions, especially in Phase II and III.

In medicine, the patients are just not all alike, nor are physicians, hospitals, or communities. Under most carefully controlled conditions, patients do as they please. So, variation is the rule to the events being studied in clinical experimentations. In the main, our results are of the form that more or fewer people respond to a new therapy than to the old one. We find tendencies, rarely laws. Once we are far from all-or-none situation measurement of uncertainty becomes important. Thus, a fundamental idea from statistics is that we must use probabilistic as well as deterministic thinking. Further the validity of any clinical experimentation depends on the manner in which the experimentation data or observations are collected, i.e. on the design and conduct of the study, as well as the manner in which the data are analyzed. Such considerations are often the areas of expertise of the statisticians.

VI

Some Statistical Designs for more Ethical Clinical Trial

Standard Fixed Size Randomized Clinical Trial: The vocabulary and methods of standard clinical trial are to be found within classical statistical "hypothesis testing" founded by Neyman and Pearson. A good elementary discussion of the statistical concepts underlying the standard type of trial can be found in Hoel (1976), and the more clinical methods have been reviewed in Feinstein (1977 and 1986). This type of trial requires a specific fixed number of patients and also demands considerable time and expense. Nevertheless, it is traditionally viewed as the "gold standard" in clinical investigation (Schaffner, 1983). A number of commentators have faced difficulties arising out of the ethical features of such a design based on fixed number of observations. It has been noted that there is no way of monitoring the results of the trial without compromising its efficiency (Clayton, 1982), (Tukey, 1977). Some investigators are further concerned that a trial may continue too long, resulting either in excess harm if the new therapy is not beneficial, or in a delay in administration of the new therapy to later patients should it prove effective. These concerns have led to development of increasingly recognized, even if not widely implemented, type of trial that still falls within the ambit of classical tradition. This kind of trial, known as *sequential trial*, arose out of wartime work on military quality control in 1940s by Abraham Wald (1947) and George Barnard (1946). In particular, the major influence on the subject has been the work of Wald (1947) related to sequential probability ratio test (SPRT).

Sequential Trial: The principal feature of a sequential procedure is a sampling scheme, which lays a rule under which one decides at each stage of sampling whether to stop or to continue sampling. This decision is being taken in the light of observations already accumulated. There are a number of different designs available under this rubric, and the interested reader may refer Armitage (1975) and Whitehead (1983). Sequential trials do not eliminate the problem of reduced statistical efficiency due to continuous monitoring of the data, though they do take this into account in the statistical calculations. Such trials make it possible to limit the harm a new substance or a technique may cause, and also may allow an efficacious new therapy to become accepted more quickly. Whitehead (1983, p. 21) puts it as follows:

> The ethical desirability of terminating a trial which shows an early advantage for one or other of the treatments is the primary motivation for the use of a technique which is called "sequential analysis" . . . In a sequential trial the decision to stop admission to the trial depends on the nature of the evidence accumulated so far. If early evidence indicates the clear superiority of one or other of the treatments, then the trial will be short, enabling an unsuccessful new treatment to be dropped or a successful one to be publicized straight away. On the other hand, if the evidence builds up without indicating a clear conclusion then the trial will be of longer duration. The sample size will thus be random variable, with a distribution depending on the true treatment difference and on the sequential design used.

Whitehead indicated that many of the types of sequential designs available

> will give sample sizes which, even when the comparison of treatments is at its most difficult, achieve typical values well below equivalent fixed sample procedures. Thus a likely reduction in patient numbers is a secondary advantage of the sequential approach. — 1983, p. 21

***Progressive Censoring Scheme (PCS)*:** A natural characteristic of clinical trials (and life-testing experimentations) is that the observations are gathered sequentially in time. Because of practical limitations (on the cost and duration of experimentation) it is not always possible to continue experimentation until all individuals responded and then to draw statistical inference. Usually the experiment is curtailed either after a specified length of time or after a prespecified proportion (or number) of individuals responded. In statistical terminology such procedures are termed respectively the truncated or censored procedures. In the truncated scheme, the duration of the experiment is prefixed, but the number of respondents is a random variable. On the other hand, in the censored case, the number of respondents is prefixed, but the duration of the experiment is a random variable. However, in most practical problems, fixed point truncation or censoring may lead to considerable loss of efficiency relative to cost. This drawback is particularly felt in exploratory studies. A too early termination of the experiment may lead to an adequately small set of observations and thus increase the risk of incorrect decision. Unnecessary prolongation of the experiment may lead to loss of valuable time with practically no extra gain in efficiency. To avoid this Chatterjee and Sen (1973) (see also Sen, 1978) introduced PCS which allows one to monitor the experiment from the beginning until a statistically valid decision (with prescribed risk) is made.

Partially Sequential Trial: In order to capitalize the best aspects of both fixed sample size and sequential procedure, Wolfe (1977) introduced partially sequential sampling scheme. In the words of Wolfe (1977) it may be mentioned that this type of partially sequential sampling procedures are particularly applicable for certain data collection setting among which the following two are important:

1. One of the samples has been previously collected and we do not wish to collect any more observations than are necessary for reaching a decision.
2. Neither samples have been collected, but one of the samples is easy and relatively inexpensive and the other is costly and/or difficult to obtain.

An example of the second type of data collection setting can be found in a real life medical problem that has been discussed by Efron (1980). There he was interested whether the easier technique ("regular") for measuring lymphocyte levels in human subject can be substituted for the difficult ("micro") one, without any loss of important information. This partially sequential scheme is based on an inverse sampling technique, where, based on random sample of fixed size from the easier/cheapest of the two treatments, a region is demarcated. The observations from the other treatment are then drawn sequentially until a previously fixed number of observations fall in the demarcated region. Data are then analyzed for decision. More recent works in this area are due to Bandyopadhyay and Chattopadhyay (1992), Bandyopadhyay and Chattopadhyay (1995) and Chattopadhyay (2002).

Adaptive Design: The classical sequential trials do not, however, resolve the ethical dilemma posed by the increasingly available information during the course of the trial. Such information may suggest that the new therapy is preferred, but prior to reaching a pre-chosen level of "statistical significance" the control will still be assigned to every other patient entering such trial. Towards finding a remedy, or at least to ameliorate this ethical difficulty, a number of researchers have proposed novel designs that assign a therapy based on the information generated by the trial to that point. They are termed as "adaptive design." Adaptive design in the clinical trial context was first formulated as solutions to optimal decision-making questions: "Which treatment is better? What sample size should be used prior to determining a "better" treatment to maximize the total number receiving the better treatment? How do we incorporate prior data or accruing data into these decisions?" The preliminary ideas can be traced back to Thompson (1933) and Robbins (1952) and led to a flurry of work in the 1960s by Anscombe (1963), Colton (1963), Zelen (1969) and Cornfield et al. (1969) among others. Perhaps the simplest of these adaptive designs is the *play-the-winner rule* originally explored by Robbins (1952) and later by Zelen (1969), in which a success on one treatment results in the next patient's assignment to the same treatment, and a failure on one treatment results in the next patient's assignment to the opposite treatment. The idea of Zelen (1969) has been modified by Wei and Durham (1978) eliminating the problem of deterministic allocation and was termed as *randomized play-the-winner* (RPW) *rule.* For dichotomized treatment responses ("success" or "failure") the RPW rule can be described through the following urn model. Start with an urn having two types of balls A and B corresponding to two treatments A and B respectively. Let "A" be the number of balls of either type. When a patient enters into a system it is assigned a treatment by drawing a ball at random (with replacement). If the response is success (or failure) we add an additional "B" number of balls of the same (or opossite) kind in the urn. The rule for given (A, B) is denoted by RPW (A, B). On an average RPW (A, B) rule allows more patients to be treated by better treatment during the time of decision-making. Zelen and Wei (1995) mentioned a recent clinical trial by Connor et. al. (1994) to evaluate the hypothesis that the antiviral therapy AZT reduces the risk of maternal-to-infant HIV transmission. A standard randomization scheme was used to obtain equal allocation to both AZT and placebo, resulting in 239 pregnant women receiving AZT and 238 receiving placebo. The end point was whether the newborn infant was HIV-negative or HIV-positive. An HIV-positive newborn could be diagnosed within 12 weeks, a newborn could be safely claimed to be HIV-negative within 24 weeks. The results of the trial were compelling: At the conclusion of the trial (which was stopped early), 60 newborns were HIV-positive in the placebo group and only 20 newborns were HIV-positive in the AZT group. However, these numbers mask the harsh reality that three times as many infants on placebo have received a death sentence by transmission of HIV from their mothers. Had they been AZT, one could presume that many would have been saved. Yao and Wei (1996) have shown that had RPW rule been used in several other trials, where actually 50-50 allocation rules have been followed, the ethical aspect could have been better preserved.

Besides RPW rule, different types of adaptive design are now there in statistical literature, like sequential maximum likelihood procedure (SMLE), doubly adaptive biased coin design (DBCD) of Eisele (1994), Drop-the-Loser (DL) rule of Ivanova (2003) among many others. A good account of different types of adaptive designs can be had from Rosenberger (1996) and Rosenberger and Lachin (2002). More recent works using adaptive design are due to Chattopadhyay (2004), Chattopadhyay and Chatterjee (2002) and Chattopadhyay and Chatterjee (2005).

VII

Concluding Remarks

Ethical ideas change and, we hope, advance over time. This increased sensitivity to ethical issues generates a wish to conduct clinical trials, which are more ethical. At the same time there are advances in statistical thinking. Computation facilities are also expanding resulting in capability of doing things differently. Patients are becoming better informed. Social context is changing. The interplay of these changes is likely to make change desirable, feasible and urgent and it is possible through a good patient-physician relationship. The statistical methods discussed in this article are neither the only ethical methods in clinical trial nor that all ethical dilemmas have been solved. There are several other methods and several other thinkings like Kadane-Sedransk-Seidenfeld (KSS) design (see Kadane, 1996), where the design starts from the objective of gathering information to resolve controversy among experts (physicians, scientists, researchers, etc.) and postulate multiple expert view of the background information that accruing data are to reconcile. These designs protect patients' welfare by restricting treatment assignments to those treatments determined to be favourable according to some one or more of the experts. In statistical community further search for development of methods for more ethical clinical trial is going on. However, this is my expectation that the discussions on the medical ethical issues in the present article will help in future for interdisciplinary group of researchers, especially, researchers from the field of medicine, statistics, law, philosophy, economics and sociology to develop further more principles and techniques for ethical experiments on human subjects.

Acknowledgement

The author is indebted to Dr. M. Chattopadhyay, Department of Philosophy, Jadavpur University, Kolkata and Prof. A. Chatterjee, Department of Statistics, University of Burdwan, West Bengal, for their encouragement for writing this article.

References

Anscombe, F.J. (1963), "Sequential Medical Trials," *Journal of the American Statistical Association*, 58, pp. 365-84.

Armitage, P. (1975), *Sequential Medical Trials*, Oxford: Blackwell.

Bacon, F. (1623), "De Augmentis Scientiarum," in J.M. Robertson, ed., *The Philosophical Works of Francis Bacon*, Reprint, 1970, New York: Books for Libraries Press, Freeport.

Bandyopadhyay, U. and G. Chattopadhyay (1992), "Inverse Sampling for Bivariate nonparametric two-sample test against restricted alternatives," *Calcutta Statistical Association Bulletin*, vol. 42, No. 167-68, pp. 221-36.

Bandyopadhyay, U. and G. Chattopadhyay (1995), "Progressive censoring under inverse sampling for nonparametric two-sample problems," *Sequential Analysis*, 14(1), pp. 1-28.

Barnard, G.A. (1946), "Sequential Tests in Industrial Statistics," *Journal of Royal Statistical Society*, Suppl., 8, pp. 1-26.

Beauchamp, T. and J. Childress (1989), *Principles of Biomedical Ethics*, 3rd edition, New York: Oxford University Press.

Beecher, H.K. (1966), "Ethics and clinical research," *The New England Journal of Medicine*, 274, pp. 1354-60.

Berkeley, G. (1752), "Further thoughts on tar-water," in Fraser, A.C. ed., *The Works of George Berkeley*, vol. 3, 1901, Oxford: Clarendon Press.

Brandt, A.M. (1978), *Racism and Research: The Case of the Tuskegee Syphilis Study*, Hastings Centre Report, 8(6), pp. 21-29.

Chatterjee, S.K. and P.K. Sen (1973), "Nonparametric testing under progressive censoring," *Calcutta Statistical Association Bulletin*, 22, p. 13.

Chattopadhyay, G. (2002), "Partially Sequential nonparametric two-sample test for ordererd categorical data," *Journal of Nonparametric Statistics*, 14(5), pp. 539-53.

Chattopadhyay, G. and A. Chatterjee (2002), "Dichotomization redundant randomized play-the-winner rule for continuous treatment responses in clinical trials," *Technical Report*, No. 02-07, Statistical Research Group, Japan: Hiroshima University, Higashi-Hiroshima.

Chattopadhyay, G. and A. Chatterjee (2005), "On a fixed point adaptation problem for ordinal clinical responses," *International Journal of Statistical Sciences*, vol. 4, pp. 25-48.

Chattopadhyay, G. (2004), "Randomized play-the-winner rule for ordered categorical data," *Communication in Statistics-Theory and Methods*, 33, 11, pp. 2683-2708.

Clayton, D. (1982), "Ethically optimized designs," *British Journal of Clinical Pharmocology*, 13, pp. 469-80.

Colton, T. (1963), "A model for selecting one of two medical treatments," *Journal of the American Statistical Association*, 58, pp. 388-400.

Connor, E.M., R. Sperling, P. Gelber, G. Kiselev, R.S. Scott, M.J. O'Sullivan, R. VarDyke, M. Bey, W. Shearer, R.L. Jacobson, E. Jiminez, E. O'neill, B. Bazin, J. Del-Fraissy, M. Culnane, R. Coombs, M. Elkins, J. Moye, P. Stratton, and J. Balsley (1994), "Reduction of maternal-infant transmission of human immunodeficiency virus type 1 with Zidovudine treatment," *New England Journal of Medicine*, 331, pp. 1173-80. (Report written for the Paediatric AIDS Clinical Trial Group Protocol 076 Study Group.)

Cornfield, J., M. Halperin and S.W. Greenhouse (1969), "An adaptive procedure for sequential clinical trials," *Journal of the American Statistical Association*, 64, pp. 759-70.

Dewey, J. and J.H. Tufts (1936), *Ethics*, revised, New York: Henry Holt.

Ebersold, L.A. (1973), "The University of Cincinnati Whole-Body Radiation Study: For Whose Benefit?" 15, *Atomic Energy*, L.J. p. 155.

Efron, B. (1980), "Which of the two measurements is better?" *Biostatistics casebook* (ed., R.G. Miller et al.), New York: John Wiley, pp. 153-70.

Eisele, J.R. (1994), "The doubly adaptive biased coin design for sequential clinical trials," *Journal of Statistical Planning and Inference,* 38, pp. 249-61.

Feinstein, A. (1977), *Clinical Biostatistics,* St. Louis: Mosby.

Feinstein, A. (1986), *Clinical Epidemiology: The Architecture of Clinical Research,* Philadelphia: Saunders.

Fried, C. (1974), *Medical Experimentation: Personal Integrity and Social Policy,* New York: Oxford University Press.

Hoel, P. (1976), *Elementary Statistics,* 4th ed., New York: John Wiley.

Ivanova, A.V. (2003), "A play-the-winner type urn design with reduced variability," *Metrika,* 58, pp. 1-13.

Jones, J.H. (1981), *Bad Blood: The Tuskegee Syphilis Experiment,* New York: The Free Press.

Kadane, J.B. (1996), *Bayesian Methods and Ethics in a Clinical Trial Design,* New York: John Wiley & Sons.

Kairys, D. (1996), "The laws of clinical testing with human subjects: Legal implications of the new and existing methodologies," in J.B. Kadane, (ed.) *Bayesian Methods and Ethics in a Clinical Trial Design,* New York: John Wiley & Sons, p. 223.

Katz, J. (1972), *Experimentation with Human Beings,* New York: Russell Sage.

Levine, R. and K. Labacqz (1979), "Some ethical considerations in clinical trials," *Clinical Pharmacology and Therapeutics,* 25, pp. 728-41.

Louis, P.C.A. (1836), *Researches on the effects of Blood-Letting* (trans.) C.G. Putnam, Boston.

Louis, P.C.A. (1834), *Essay on Clinical Instruction* (trans.), P. Martin, London.

Mitford, J. (1974), *Kind and Usual Punishment,* pp. 151-84.

Pappworth, M.H. (1967), *Human Guinea Pigs,* Boston: Beacon Press.

Rawls, J. (1971), *A Theory of Justice,* Cambridge: Harvard University Press.

Robbins, H. (1952), "Some aspects of the sequential design of experiments," *Bulletin of the American Mathematical Society,* 58, pp. 527-35.

Rosenberger, W.F. (1996), "New Directions in Adaptive Design," *Statistical Science,* 13, 2, pp. 137-49.

Rosenberger, W.F. and J.M. Lachin (2002), *Randomization in Clinical Trials-Theory and Practice,* New York: John Wiley.

Ross, W.D. (1930), *The Right and the Good*, Oxford: Clarendon Press.

Schaffner, K.F. (1996), "Ethically optimizing clinical trials, in Kadane," in J.B. (ed.), *Bayesian methods and Ethics in a Clinical Trial Design*, New York: John Wiley & Sons, p. 19.

Schaffner, K.F. (1987), "Causation in Medicine and the Law," in *Medical Innovation and Bad Outcomes: Legal, Social and Ethical Responses*, Ann Arbor, MI: Health Administration Press, pp. 71-99.

Schaffner, K.F. (1983), *Clinical Trials: The validation theory and therapy, physics, philosophy and psychoanalysis*, L. Laudan and R. Cohen (eds.) Dordrecht, Reidel, pp. 191-208.

Sen, P.K. (1978), "Nonparametric repeated significance tests," in P.R. Krishnaiah, ed., *Developments in Statistics*, vol. 1, New York: Academic Press, p. 227.

Thompson, W.R. (1933), "On the likelihood that one unknown probability exceeds another in the view of the evidence of the two samples," *Biometrika*, 25, pp. 275-94.

Tukey, J. (1977), "Some thoughts on clinical trials, especially problems of multiplicity," *Science*, 198, pp. 679-83.

Wald, A. (1947), *Sequential Analysis*, New York: John Wiley.

Wei, L.J. and S. Durham (1978), "The randomized play-the-winner rule in medical trials," in *Journal of the American Statistical Association*, 73, pp. 830-43.

Whitehead, J. (1983), *The design and analysis of sequential clinical trials*, New York: Halsted Press (Wiley).

Wolfe, D.A. (1977), "On a class of partially sequential two-sample test procedures," in *Journal of the American Statistical Association*, 72, p. 202.

Yao, Q. and L.J. Wei (1996), "Play the winner for phase II/III clinical trials," *Statistics in Medicine*, 15, pp. 2413-23.

Zelen, M. (1969), "Play-the-winner rule and the controlled clinical trial," in *Journal of the American Statistical Association*, 64, pp. 131-46.

Zelen, M. and L.J. Wei (1955), Foreward in *Adaptive Designs* (N. Flournoy and W.F. Rosenberger, eds.), IMS, Hayward, CA.

12

Medicine and Law
In the Perspective of Physician-Patient Relationship

Malay Kumar Basu

GONE are the days when the physician-patient relationship was marked by deepest regard, extreme cordiality and unbounded faith. A family physician used to command unflinching respect and total devotion from the patient and his relations who used to regard him as their friend, philosopher and guide. Hardly there was an incident of violence in the event of any patient not responding to the treatment of the doctor or even the patient having been a victim of the doctor's wrong treatment. Hardly his relatives or friends held the doctor responsible or pounced upon him in vengeance. But this classical concept of Doctor-Patient relationship has unfortunately been given a complete burial today due to the result of cumulative interaction of mass media, medical development and legislation. There has been a huge advancement in medical technology and technical competence which has led to an unprecedented increase in the level of people's awareness and expectations. As in all other spheres of life, the people who receive medical treatment have begun to assert their rights. Thus "today's patient is more conscious of his rights, more informed, educated and poised to change the face of health care concept altogether."

Law is a product of social need. As the society progresses, in order to cope with the changing pattern of society the Statute Book has to undergo a corresponding change failing which there will be created a vacuum which may have serious, disconcerting effect on the harmonious growth of the society. The Laws on Medicine in the perspective of Doctor-Patient relationship also owe their origin and development to such changing needs of the society throughout the different ages since time immemorial. Even as far back as in 1000 BCE there was no dearth of consciousness on the part of the people of our country about the importance of enforicng certain checks and balances on the activities of a doctor dealing with the lives of the multitude. As we find, a host of duties and responsibilities were cast on the doctors in the form of what is called Caraka's oath. Similar practices flourished during the Greek Civilization when oaths of the like nature used to be administered to the medical professionals on the eve of their starting the noble profession. This has been popularly known as Hippocratic oath. Display of utmost vigilance on the part of the Legislators of all ages to control the conduct of the medical man is quite understandable. The noble profession has been gradually undergoing drastic changes in its journey towards thorough commercialization since the ancient times when it commanded deepest respect from the people due to its philanthropic character imbued with missionary zeal. As a matter of fact under the Roman Law the services of a physician were strictly honorary and under the common Law of England a physician was presumed to attend to his patient for an honorarium. But today all-pervading element of commerce is fast changing the complexion of doctor-patient relationship and in the result a series of legislations, rules and regulations have been emerging since the last century to provide safeguards against the lapses and laches, faults and failures indulged in by the professionals in this noble vocation. Nothing hereinbefore has become a more burning topic in the legal domain or in the social parlour than the expression, "Medical Negligence," which has gained so much currency and controversy that a series of landmark judgements had to be pronounced by the highest court of our country to set the anomalies at rest. These decisions of the Apex Court have now come to govern the subject.

The modern Law on Medicine is to be understood in its various remifications. The principles governing medical negligence of a physician, surgeon or a dentist are lying scattered in the Civil, Criminal and Consumer Courts of our country. The chief object of the Medical Law is to regulate the medical profession and the administration of hospitals, by spelling out the criteria of reasonable care and competence and standard of professional knowledge and skill, and also by spelling out the various duties of a doctor — like duties to the patient, duties to the public, duties to the law enforcers, duties to each other, duties not to violate professional ethics, duties not to do anything illegal, etc. Such laws further dwell upon the subjects like duties of the patient, doctor-patient contract, professional secrets, necessity of consent in medical treatment, various forms of consent like express consent, implied consent, informed consent, proxy consent, or situations where consent may not be obtained.

Let us enumerate and take a glimpse from some of the major statutes in their chronological order which were enacted by our legislature from time to time for serving the above purposes.

The Bengal Medical Act, 1914

In a word the Bengal Medical Act, 1914 was to provide for registration of medical practitioners in this State. Under this Act the West Bengal Medical Council was established. The Constitution of the Council, its functions and other particulars have been spelt out in different Sections of this Act. Provisions have also been laid down herein for maintaining a register where the names of the registered practitioners who possess the requisite qualifications are to be entered (Section 17). The Council has also been given the power to direct removal of the names of any such practitioners from the register in case he/she is sentenced by any Criminal Court for committing any non-bailable offence or if the Council after having held its own enquiry finds him or her guilty of any infamous conduct in any professional respect (Section 25). This enactment was perhaps the first of its kind in the matter of regulating the conduct of those adopting the profession of medical practice and to check entry of unqualified persons called quacks in this field. In the schedule of this Act, the qualifications which will entitle an applicant to registration have been spelt out.

Indian Medical Degrees Act, 1916

The second statute on the subject in British India worth mentioning is the Indian Medical Degrees Act, 1916 which was enacted with a view to restricting the rights of various provincial authorities to issue degrees and diplomas in the field of medicine and surgery with the purpose of ensuring that such degrees or diplomas are not conferred upon unqualified persons. This Act has specified certain authorities as competent to issue the degrees and diplomas and has spelt out penal provisions to punish those persons who falsely assume any medical title.

Indian Medical Council Act, 1956

The law that next deserves mention was a product of the legislature of Independent India. It is the Indian Medical Council Act, 1956. Its object was to make provision for reconstitution of the Medical Council of India and maintenance of a medical register for matters connected therewith. Under this Act the words like "medicine," "recognized medical qualifications," etc. were defined. Thus, it has been stated that "medicine" means modern scientific medicine in all its branches and includes surgery and obstetrics but excludes veterinary medicine and surgery. U/S 10A of this Act no person can establish a medical college or no medical college can open a new higher course of study or training or can increase its admission capacity in any course of study or training except with the prior permission of the Central Government. In this way this legislation also was aimed at keeping the medical profession free from being polluted by the entry of people who did not receive proper and prescribed medical education or training and at whose hands patients' lives might be endangered if they were allowed to treat them.

The importance of this Act, however, lies in its incorporating a special provision enabling the Medical Council to make regulations providing for the standards of professional conduct and etiquette and code of ethics to be observed by medical practitioners [vide section 33 (m)]. On the basis of this provision Regulations have also been framed laying down *inter alia* a code of ethics to be followed by a medical practitioner, viz. The IMC (Professional Conduct, Etiquette and Ethics) Regulations, 2002. According to the Regulation, each applicant at the time of his registration is to be given by the Registrar concerned a copy of a "Declaration" containing certain promises which he will have to read out and agree to abide by. These promises are quoted below:

1. I solemnly pledge myself to consecrate my life to the service of humanity.
2. Even under threat, I will not use my medical knowledge contrary to the laws of humanity.
3. I will maintain the utmost respect for human life from the time of conception.
4. I will not permit consideration of religion, nationality, race, party politics or social standing to intervene between my duty and my patient.
5. I will practise my profession with conscience and dignity.
6. The health of my patient will be my first consideration.
7. I will respect the secrets which are confided in me.
8. I will give to my teachers the respect and gratitude which is their due.
9. I will maintain, by all means in my power, the honour and noble traditions of medical profession.
10. My colleagues will be my brothers.

The second part of the code spells out certain general principles, which are as follows:

CHARACTER OF THE PHYSICIAN

The prime object of the medical profession is to render service to humanity; reward of financial gain is a subordinate consideration. Whosoever chooses this profession, assumes the obligation to conduct himself in accordance with its ideals. A physician should be an upright man, instructed in the "art of healing." He must keep himself pure in character and be diligent in caring for the sick. He should be modest, sober, patient, prompt to do his whole duty without anxiety; pious without going so far as superstition, conducting himself with propriety in his profession and in all the actions of his life.

THE PHYSICIAN'S RESPONSIBILITY

The principal objective of the medical profession is to render service to humanity with full respect for the dignity of man. Physicians should merit the confidence of patients entrusted to their care, rendering to each a full measure of service and devotion. Physicians should try continuously to improve medical knowledge and skill and should make available to their patients and colleagues the benefits of their professional attainments. The physician should practise methods of healing founded on scientific basis and should not associate professionally with anyone who violates this principle. The honoured ideals of the medical profession imply that the responsibilities of the physician extend not only to individuals but also to society.

PAYMENT FOR PROFESSIONAL SERVICES

The ethical physician, engaged in the practice of medicine, limits the sources of his income received from professional activities to services rendered to the patient. A physician should announce his fees or remunerations before rendering service and not after the operation or when the treatment is under way. Remuneration received for such services should be in the form and amount specifically announced to the patient at the time the service is rendered. It is unethical to enter into a contract of "no cure no payment. Physician rendering service on behalf of the State should refrain from anticipating or accepting any consideration."

From the standpoint of patient-physician relationship, such inclusion of this code of ethics assumes particular significance inasmuch as any violation of any of such prescriptions will entail legal consequence since it will constitute medical negligence for which the doctor will have to account for.

Chapter 7 of the said Regulations 2002 enumerates some of the acts or omissions on the part of a medical practitioner which constitute misconduct rendering him or her liable for disciplinary action:

(a) violation of any of the regulations promulgated,

(b) not maintaining of medical records of the indoor patients,

(c) refusing to provide the medical records within 72 hours when the patient or his/her authorized representative makes a request for it,

(d) not displaying the registration number accorded to him by the State Medical Council or the Medical Council of India in his clinic, prescriptions, certificates, etc. issued by him,

(e) adultery or improper conduct,

(f) conviction by Court of Law,

(g) sex determination test,

(h) not obtaining consent in writing from the guardians or relatives of the patient,

(i) using touts or agents for procuring patients, and

(j) claiming himself/herself to be a Specialist without having a special qualification in the concerned branch.

Under Chapter 8, disciplinary action and punishment have been provided for being awarded in case of such instances of professional misconduct by the appropriate Medical Council which may direct removal of the name of the delinquent registered practitioner from the Register either for a temporary, specified period or permanently.

As we have pointed out above, such duties and responsibilities were entrusted upon the medical practitioners even in the ancient era in some form or the other. The famous "Caraka's oath" which was in vogue in 1000 BCE used to be administered to the medical students by the teacher in the form of instructions given in the presence of the Sacred Fire, Brahmanas and Physicians. These were as follows:

> Thou shalt be free from envy, not cause another's death, and pray for the welfare of all creatures. Day and night thou shalt not desert a patient, nor commit adultery, be modest in thy attire and appearance, not to be drunkard or sinful, while entering a patients's house, be accompanied by a person known to the patient. The peculiar customs of the patient's household shall not be made public.

Then in 460 BCE under the Greek civilization, Hippocratic oath gained currency. A person willing to enter into the medical profession had to swear by the names of the gods and goddesses and take the following oath —

- "To consider dear to me as my parents him who taught me this art;
- to live in common with him and if necessary to share my goods with him;
- to look upon his children as my own brothers, to teach them this art if they so desire without fee or written promise;
- to impart to my sons and the sons of the master who taught me and the disciples who have enrolled

themselves and have agreed to the rules of the profession, but to these alone, the precepts and the instruction.

- I will prescribe regimen for the good of my patients according to my ability and my judgement and never do harm to anyone.
- To please no one will I prescribe a deadly drug, nor give advice which may cause his death.
- Nor I will give a woman a pessary to procure abortion.
- But I will preserve the purity of my life and my art. I will not cut for stone, even for patients in whom the disease is manifest; I will leave this operation to be performed by practitioners (specialists in this art).
- In every house where I come I will enter only for the good of my patients, keeping myself far from all intentional ill-doing and all seduction, and especially from the pleasures of love with women or with men, be they free or slaves.
- All that may come to my knowledge in the exercise of my profession or outside of my profession or in daily commerce with men, which ought not to be spread abroad, I will keep secret and will never reveal.
- If I keep this oath faithfully may I enjoy my life and practise my art, respected by all men and in all times, but if I swerve from it or violate it may the reverse be my lot."

In the modern era the necessity of administration of such oaths to a new entrant in the medical profession was felt by the World Medical Association which proclaimed its resolution in 1968 popularly called Geneva Declaration on the reasoning that it is the mission of the medical Doctor to safeguard the health of the people and his or her knowledge and conscience are dedicated to the fulfilment of this mission. These oaths are as follows:

(As amended at Sydney, 1968)

At the time of being admitted as a member of the medical profession:

- I will solemnly pledge myself to consecrate my life to the service of humanity;
- I will give to my teachers the respect and gratitude which is their due;
- I will practise my profession with conscience and dignity;
- The health of my patient will be my first consideration;
- I will respect the secrets which are confided in me, even after the patient has died;
- I will maintain by all the means in my power the honour and the noble traditions of the medical profession;
- My colleagues will be my brothers;
- I will not permit considerations of religion, nationality; race, party politics or social standing to intervene between my duty and my patient;
- I will maintain the utmost respect for human life from the time of conception. Even under threat I will not use my medical knowledge contrary to the laws of humanity; and
- I make these promises solemnly, freely and upon my honour.

[See P-9 (a) to 9 (e)]

But the above legislations have not been able to produce the desired result. Greed for money and erosion of values on the part of the doctors have caused serious disconcerting effect on the patient-physician relationship. Such a turmoil has given birth to still another piece of legislation which has ultimately come to govern the subject. This is called the Consumer Protection Act, 1986 which was intended to provide for better protection of the interests of the consumers. But this welfare legislation was kept away from the arena of the medical practitioner for a considerable period on the plea that medical service did not fall within the mischief of the definition of the word "Service." It was in 1995 that the Apex Court of our country had to pass a landmark judgement directing inclusion of the service rendered by a physician to his patient as a service which would fall within the "category of services" as defined under the Consumer Protection Act, 1986. Since this judgement has been pronounced, the doctors all over the country have been subjected to the provisions of the Consumer Protection Act, 1986 and thus this legislation has practically brought about a revolution in the legal history concerning the medical world. Under the Consumer Protection Act in Section 2 (o), the word "Service" has been defined as follows:

> 'Service' means service of any description which is made available to potential users and includes facilities in connection with banking, financing, insurance, transport, processing, supply of electrical or other energy, board or lodging or both, housing construction, entertainment, amusement or briefing of news or other information, but does not include rendering of any service free of charge or under a contract of personal service.

For a long time people were under the impression that the relationship between a medical practitioner and the patient is one of trust and confidence and therefore, it was in the nature of a contract of personal service and that being so, the service rendered by the medical practitioners to their patients was not "Service" U/S 2(1) (o) of the Act. This very argument was advanced before the Supreme Court in Indian Medical Association vs. V.P. Shantha. After thorough and careful consideration of the points urged in this case, the Hon'ble Court has held that it is no doubt true that the relationship between a medical practitioner and a patient carries within it a certain degree of mutual confidence and trust and, therefore, the services rendered by the medical practitioner can be regarded as services of a personal nature. But since there is no relationship of master-and-servant between the doctor and the patient, the contract between the medical practitioner and his patient cannot be treated as a contract of personal service, but is a contract for services, and the service rendered by the medical practitioner to his patient under such a contract is not covered by the exclusionary part of the definition of service contained in Section 2(1) (o) of the Act (vide decision reported in (1995) 6 Supreme Court cases 651 corresponding to: (1995), 3 CPJ 1 (SC). In V.P. Nair vs. Cosmopolitan Hospital (P) Ltd. reported in (1991) 2 CPJ 444 (Kerala) it has been held that there is, in a general sense, a personal element in the medical officer's service to their clients, but we do not think that they can be called personal service and although a medical officer's service may occasionally or marginally be called personal service, it would be incorrect to describe it as personal service, because personal service stems from a master-and-servant relationship.

Regarding what constitutes medical negligence there has been a plethora of rulings of the Supreme Court as well as the

National Consumer Commission which have by this time settled the position. In the above-mentioned judgement of the Apex Court, it has been observed that unless facts and circumstances unmistakably point to negligence or professional misconduct of a medical practitioner without the aid of an expert, there are practical difficulties in linking the injury sustained with the medical treatment. It is now a settled position that a doctor, who has taken the responsibility of a patient, has threefold duties to discharge, namely a duty of care in deciding whether to undertake the case, a duty of care in deciding what treatment to give and a duty of care in the administration of the treatment (vide the above-mentioned reported decision in Indian Medical Association vs. V.P. Shantha & Others). A breach of any of these duties gives to the patient a right of action for negligence. "A person who holds himself out ready to give medical advice and treatment impliedly undertakes that he has possessed all skill and knowledge for the purpose. Such a person when consulted by a patient owes him such duties. The practitioner must bring to his task a reasonable degree of skill and knowledge and must exercise a reasonable degree of care. Neither the very highest nor a very low degree of care and competence judged in the light of the particular circumstances of each case is what the law requires. The doctor no doubt has a discretion in choosing treatment which he proposes to give to the patient and such discretion is relatively ampler in cases of emergency." The dictionary meaning of the word "negligence" is omission to do something which a reasonable man guided by those ordinary considerations which ordinarily regulate human affairs would do or the doing of something which a reasonable and prudent man would not do. Under the law of tort also, this is the meaning of negligence that it is a breach of duty caused by omission to do something which a reasonable man would do or doing something which a prudent and reasonable man would not do. Thus this definition of the word "negligence" involves three constituents:

1. A legal duty to exercise due care;
2. A breach of the duty; and
3. Consequential damages.

The decision in the case of Golum vs. Fiern Hospital Management Committee reported in (1957) 2 All England Reporter 118, it was held by Justice McNair that the test is the standard of the ordinary by skilled man exercising and professing to have the special skill. The man need not possess the highest expert skill; it is well established law that it is sufficient if he exercises the ordinary skill of an ordinary competent man exercising that particular art. In the case of medical man, negligence means failure to act in accordance with the standards of reasonably competent medical men at the time of treatment of a patient. There may be one or more perfectly proper standards and if he conforms to one of those proper standards, then he is not negligent.

A question arose as to whether error of judgement constitutes an act of negligence on the part of a physician. In Spring Meadows Hospital vs. Harjot Ahluwallia, the Supreme Court has settled the position by observing that the "true position" is that an error of judgement may or may not be negligent; it depends on the nature of the error. If it is one that would not have been made by a reasonably competent professional man professing to have the "standard and type of skill," the defendant held himself out as having acted with ordinary care, then it is negligence. If, on the other hand, it is an error that such a man acting with ordinary care might have made, then it is not negligence. Gross medical mistake will always result in a finding of negligence. Use of wrong drug or wrong gas during the course of anaesthesia will frequently lead to the imposition of liability and in some situations even the principles of *res ipsa loquitur* can be applied. Even delegation of responsibility to another may amount to negligence in certain circumstances. A consultant could be negligent where he delegates the responsibility to his junior with the knowledge that the junior was incapable of performing his duties properly.

After the medical service rendered by a doctor has been included within the ambit and scope of the Consumer Protection Act, the Consumer Courts have been flooded with cases complaining about negligence on the part of the doctors while rendering medical treatment to the patients and these courts are to apply various settled principles to ascertain whether in the light of such maxims the doctor can be said to be at fault. In such cases the remedy that is sought by the complainants is generally compensation for the loss or damage caused to them in consequence of the negligent act of the said doctor. Thus the emergence of this law has gone a long way in re-defining the patient-physician relationship and in curbing the excesses which the latter used to exert in the recent years posing a threat to the harmonious relationship between the two. The word "deficiency" has been defined under the Consumer Protection Act as meaning fault, imperfection, short-coming or inadequacy.

However, cases against the doctors for their negligence used to be filed even before the coming into force of the Consumer Protection Act and this was under the law of torts before the ordinary Civil Courts. Doctors providing free or paid services were liable to be proceeded against for claiming compensation under the general law of tort for their negligence in treatment and also under the criminal law.

Maybe, the Consumer Protection Act has been of recent origin in order to provide speedy, inexpensive and simple remedy to a consumer (that is, to the patient or his relative) and this remedy is in addition to the already existing remedies, namely remedies under the civil laws and remedies under the criminal law. In this regard, the Apex Court has made the following observations:

> By holding that medical practitioners fall within the purview of the Consumer Protection Act, no change is brought about in the substantive law governing claims for compensation on the ground of negligence and the principles which applied to determination of such a claim before the Civil Court would equally apply to consumer disputes before the consumer disputes redressal agencies under the Act.

There are other landmark judgements of the Supreme Court as well as the National Commission determining various questions touching upon the significance of the expression "medical negligence" and the physician-patient relationship. Thus it has been held that negligence is the breach of a duty caused by the omission to do something which a prudent and reasonable man would do or doing something which a prudent and reasonable man would not do. In Vinitha Ashoke vs. Laxmi Hospital & Others, the question arose before the Supreme Court whether termination of pregnancy on the basis of evidence on record without performing ultra sonography for determining whether Appellant had ectopic pregnancy or not amounted to medical negligence. It was held that when two views were possible on whether ultra sonography would be able to identify ectopic pregnancy or not, no negligence can be attributed to doctors in not adopting it [1 (2002) CPJ 4(SC)]. On a number of occasions questions have arisen before the Consumer Courts as to whether expert evidence could be essentially required to be adduced by the Complainant for proving the alleged negligence on the part of the doctor. It has been held by different courts that expert evidence would be required in cases where the principle of *res ipsa loquitur* is not applicable. It has also been an established principle that where medical negligence cannot be proved by the Complainant, no liability can be fastened on the doctor or the hospital. Many a times this question has tormented the courts whether error of judgement should be treated as an act of negligence. The answer to this question has been given by the Apex Court as well as the National Commission in a number of judgements observing as follows:

> In such respects the guiding principle that has been enunciated is to the effect that the test will be to see if he or she has been proved to be guilty of such failure as no doctor of ordinary skill could be guilty of it acting with reasonable care (Dr. Sr. Lowie vs. Smt. K. Pathumma reported in 1993(1) CRP 422 NC).

In Sir Gangaram Hospital vs. D.P. Vandari & Others reported in 1992(2) CPJ 397, the National Consumer Commission, New Delhi held that there was no negligence or deficiency on the part of the hospital in not transferring the patient to I.C.U. on account of non-availability of vacant bed in the I.C.U. And it was also not negligence or deficiency on the part of the hospital merely on account of their omission to inform the relative of the patient to shift the patient to some other hospital if they so chose in view of the non-availability of vacant bed in the I.C.U. In Harjot Ahluwalia vs. Spring Meadows Hospital reported in 1997(2) CPJ 98, the National Commission held that the hospital was responsible for the acts of its employees and they are liable for the consequence of their negligence and was liable to pay damages to the extent of Rs. 1,00,000/- and

Rs. 5,000/- as compensation for the mental agony suffered by the Complainant and also Rs. 1,000/- as cost. This judgement of the National Commission was affirmed by the Supreme Court in its judgement reported in 1998(3) CPJ 1. In another case the Commission found a surgeon negligent when he during operation left a foreign body namely a gauze piece inside the wound and closed the operated area. Sinus developed as a result causing pain and pus oozing out. The Court awarded compensation of Rs. 40,000/- and odd towards the cost of treatment and Rs. 25,000/- on account of mental and physical agony and also Rs. 3,000/- as cost.

In this way, there have been thousands of cases in different courts all over the country where the fault or negligence on the part of the doctors is properly dealt with under the law. Thereby, constant pressure is being exerted upon the community of doctors treating the patients. Such case laws have thus gone a long way in providing suitable checks and balances on the behaviour pattern and treatment method adopted by them. Due to shortage of space such cases cannot be discussed at length. However we may only mention a few of the leading judgements which have gained currency. For example, we can cite the case of Calcutta Medical Research Institute vs. Bimalesh Chatterjee & Others [1999 (1) CPR 3] wherein the National Commission held that where the State Commission placed reliance upon a certificate issued by a doctor who was not a Specialist in the field and could not be treated as an expert, such opinion could not form the basis of the findings of the State Commission holding the Out-patient doctor negligent. The case of Charan Singh vs. Healing Touch Hospital & Others also deserves mention wherein the National Commission came to the finding that the anaesthetist followed the norm as per accepted medical procedure and settled position on the subject and therefore he could not be held guilty of any negligence. Mention may also be made of the case law reported in Consumer Protection Council & Others vs. Dr. S. Sundaram [1997(2) CPR 162 (NCDRC)] wherein the Apex Consumer Court held that the Out-patient doctor who was a highly qualified pathologist holding M.D. degree and recipient of several gold and silver medals for her papers and was willing to part with her slides for re-examination by another pathologist, it could not be said that the pathological report given by her suffered from any infirmity due to negligence or fault on the part of this expert. We shall discuss other such case laws of importance at the appropriate time.

It should not be forgotten that just as a doctor has a large number of duties and obligations towards his patient to be performed and discharged for their proper treatment and care, the patients or their relatives also have corresponding duties to be observed towards their physician. If both the sides properly and sincerely attend to such norms, then the chances of conflict or confrontation between the two will be minimized and the world will be a better place to live in. As in all the spheres of life, revival of the ethical values and imparting of moral education can in the ultimate analysis bring about a solution.

13

Status of Patients and Physicians in Indian Scenario

Its Improvement for Delivery of Better Health Care

Bansi Badan Mukhopadhyay

MORBIDITY is one of the widespread causes of human deprivation and economic insecurity. It affects not only the patients and those who depend on them for their subsistence, but also other people of the society, in so far as the threat of disease and associated morbidity affects the quality of life. A well developed public health system is a contribution to the improvement of quality of life. India has poor health achievements compared to the developed nations.

The mismatch between the resources spent on health and achievements is due to poor functioning of the public health care system especially in rural areas. In some States, this system is little more than a collection of deserted primary health centres, dirty dispensaries, unmotivated doctors and over-crowded and chaotic hospitals. Many studies have indicated that the rural health care system in some States stresses overwhelming priority to family planning at the cost of the essential health care services. To the political parties, the social security and public health issues have little place in party programmes and electoral debates. Little time is being spent on real issues such as undernutrition, illiteracy, unemployment, ill health, substandard delivery of health care services and their root causes. In India literacy is not a prerequisite of effective participation in the political process, but it is definitely a useful tool of successfully active involvement in all aspects of prosperity of the country. Would the country be more literate, the disadvantaged sections of population would successfully put their demand of better health care services and other associated needs on the political agenda. The need of basic education and development of appropriate information, education and communications (IEC) strategy is of utmost importance. The need for forming more effective political organization of deprived sections is essential and this will help development of a good effective physician-patient relationship after being confronted by both. The present issue is a very relevant and felt-need issue and deserves indepth discussions and ethical considerations.

India is a Union of 28 States and 7 Union Territories. Each State has developed its health system according to its own need. However, the basic planning is made by the Government of India and the States try to implement it. In India, majority of the patients receive the management and treatment of their ailments in the public health system which caters its services in the Government Hospitals and health centres free of cost/ at a nominal charge. The others seek health care services at the private sectors on paying considerable charges. The infrastructural facilities are not alike in the two systems with unlike quality and quantity of patient care. A patient-friendly hospital is an institutional mechanism through which patients with health problems are identified in a timely and systematic manner, attended to, examined, investigated and/or treated promptly at an appropriate health care facility. A hospital is a medico-social organization where patients are the health seekers, doctors and supportive staff are the health providers and health manager is the health administration.

In India the health system is chained with a well connected network from the community level to tertiary care. The system of health services is carried out by the following agencies.

PUBLIC AGENCIES

- Primary Health Centre/Sub Centre
- Hospitals:Rural/Subdivision/District/Specialist Teaching
- Health Insurance schemes: Employees State Insurance Scheme/Central Government Health Scheme
- Other agencies: Defence hospital; Railway hospital

PRIVATE AGENCIES

- Private hospitals
- Polyclinics
- Nursing Homes
- Dispensaries
- General practitioners' clinics

INDIGENOUS SYSTEM OF MEDICINE

- Āyurvedic & Siddha
- Unani
- Homoeopathy
- Unregistered practitioners

VOLUNTARY HEALTH AGENCIES: NGOs
VERTICAL HEALTH PROGRAMMES

Time to time National Health Programmes are held mainly in the hospitals where interaction between patient-physician and management takes place. An improved patient care depends on the joint responsibility and collaborative activity of the three systems. Each component indirectly and jointly can contribute effectively towards the delivery of quality patient care. An attempt is made to discuss the role of patient, physician and management for providing better health care delivery.

HOSPITAL

Hospital is an integral part of a social and medical organization whose function is to provide for the population, the complete health care, both curative and preventive and whose out-patient services reach out to the family in its home environment. The hospital is also a centre for training of health workers and for Biosocial Research.

ORGANIZATIONAL STRUCTURE OF A HOSPITAL

A hospital has multiple functions as listed below:

Functions

Curative — OPD/In patient/Emergency/ Referral

Preventive — Prophylactic services, sentinel centre

Promotive — Family planning services, health education services

Rehabilitative

Educational

Medico-legal

Research

Training

HOSPITAL MANAGEMENT BOARD

It acts as a bridge between hospital and community. It comprises people representing various interest groups to look into the hospital situation for its development and preserves the right of flexibility which is essential to meet the changing situation and environment and accordingly grow.

Role of Management Board

- Formulation of hospital policies
- Recommending needed resources for improved services
- Advising State Government for development and expansion
- Establishing liaison between hospital and community
- Fixing accountabilities among departments and or staff
- Reviewing client satisfaction

Different committees have been set up for a hospital to look after the different activities and for close coordination. Integration among different committees is essential.

- Administration Improvement Committee
- Consultative Committee on Patient Care
- Referral System Committee
- Medical Record Committee
- Purchase Committee
- Budget Reallocation Committee
- Engineering and Maintenance Committee
- Hospital Waste Disposal Committee

- Infection Control Committee
- Medical Audit, Utilization and Review Committee
- Emergency and Accident Services Committee

A hospital has three distinct sectors from the point of view of its management, namely the *service providers*, the *management* and the *health seekers (consumers)*.

> *Hospital*: Social organization
> *Service providers*: Clinicians and other staff
> *Management*: Hospital Administrators — Medical Superintendent and its supportive staff.

Systematic interplay and interaction between providers, consumers and administrators is essential for smooth functioning of the hospital.

To health seekers, the hospital is a place to receive care. For providers, the hospital is a place to work for the patients. For management, the hospital is a multidimensional organization embracing patient care, facility maintenance, custodial and food service activities.

The ultimate output of the hospital services is the patient care which is the product of team work. Doctor is the leader of the patient care team and paraprofessionals are the team members and the supportive staff are the other staff related with administration. In majority of cases there does not arise any serious problem but in case of any imbalance among the three sectors, conflict arises and this needs coordinated decision for tackling the problem.

The three systems, being interrelated and interdependent, must be managed and coordinated with maximum effectiveness, so as to direct and facilitate smooth performance of activities. In meeting this social responsibility the hospital administrators have to satisfy not only the patients but also the clinicians, nurses, technicians and other staff. This is achieved by adopting openness in communication and building mutual trust. Hospital administrators are responsible for solving a wide variety of management problems, and medical officers are responsible for patient care and health care. These two seemingly distinct areas of activity overlap, resulting into conflicts. These conflicts have to be avoided by effective inter- personnel communication.

The situation can be eased by integration of clinicians and administrators, their availability and attention to the distressed and through the activity of different committees/working groups where face to face communication will cut down the red tapism and biases to a great extent.

Interface between management and clinicians		
Input ⟶	**Process ⟶**	**Output**
M-Man M-Machine M-Material M-Money M-Method	P-Planning O-Organization S-Staffing D-Directing Co-ordination R-Reporting B-Budgetting E-Evaluation	P-Patient care Q-Quantity Q-Quality C-Consumer Satisfaction T-Teaching R-Research

The great challenge is one of co-ordination. If a sizeable portion is dissatisfied, the system will break down. The common mass (patients) expect hospitals to give tender, loving care to every patient everyday. Each hospital has a "personality" of its own — a tempo of work and an emotional atmosphere peculiar to a given hospital, its traditions, its community of staff and patients. The nature of staff relationship will influence the staff-patient relationship and consequently the outcome of therapy/the patient care.

The hospital system may broadly be seen as consisting of the following major systems:

- Medical care system
- Nursing care
- Ancillary system — central sterilization supplying department, infection control, cleanliness, dietary services, etc.
- Management support system — hospital information system, personnel system, logistic and supply system
- Teaching and Research Services

Goals of a modern hospital: To provide the following services:

- Patient care
- Provide primary health care to the neighbouring community
- Provide support to Primary Health Centres and act as referral centre
- Sentinel centre and to help study epidemiological measures of control
- Provide in-service training in technical aspects
- Provide diagnostic support to PHC/CHC
- Network of different medical care institutions and agents of same and of different systems of medicine

To impose the following **values**:

- Health as a value
- Focus prevention, use of appropriate technology, community involvement and multisectoral approach
- Strengthening of co-ordination through improved exchange of information collected through passive surveillance
- Value of information and feed-back

Need of adopting managerial process which is a composite process of planning and programming.

Managerial process:

- Formulation of hospital policies and setting priorities
- Preparation of programmes
- Preferential allocation of budget
- Implementation strategies and hospital service plans
- Monitoring and evaluation of patient care system
- Maintain quality of services
- Improve quality of referral care

To keep vigilance on physical environment of hospital.

Physical Environment:

- Facilities and space
- Materials and equipment
- Consultation rooms for specialist services
- Organizational structure with horizontal and vertical pathways of communication between staff
- Distribution and control of equipment and materials, at different service points

- To improve inter-personnel environment
- To take help of appropriate technology
- To maintain interface between various units

It is not enough for the hospital to be involved in the patient care alone. It must understand the Primary Health Care and its values and components and its organization to provide it.

Every hospital should evaluate from time to time the quality of services rendered. In this regard, hospital should formulate the Quality Assurance Programme (QAP) which is the delivery of relevant and effective medical care in accordance with the standards.

Medical Audit (M.A.)

It is the official examination and verification of accounts or dealings. M.A. acts as a stimulus to the practice of scientific medicine and provides mechanism of in-built check on the professional performance in the hospital. For that purpose the essential ingredient is the Medical Records on the basis of which Medical Audit can be undertaken.

Thus M.A. is the process of evaluation of medical care in retrospect through analysis of medical records.

PROCESS OF M.A.

Retrospective: Comprising the analysis of the records of the discharged patients.

- Finding out deficiencies, errors, omissions and commissions on these
- Study the inventory of the drug
- Study the ward returns

Prospective: Group of patients suffering from a common cause to be followed up and studied in respect of diagnosis, management and prognosis.

Evaluation: For evaluation of the quality of services of patient care, the hospital authority should examine the following component of services:

- Assessment of patient satisfaction from the complaint register of the patient
- Examining carefully the ward returns

Suggestions for improvement of hospital services:

It is necessary to form a Quality Control Circle (QCC) comprising 7-12 persons who will have a close look on the following:

- Improving quality of medical care
- Reducing employee turnover
- Improving employee morale
- Greater efficiency of operations
- More effective scheduling
- Reduced absenteeism
- Improved communications
- More accurate cost allocation
- Reduced costs of patient care delivery
- Improved nurse-physician relations
- Improved diet
- Improved cleanliness
- Improved surveillance system

India is a vast country with the second largest population in the world. The current population is estimated at about 110 crore. For serving such a large population the current network has been planned. As on 31st March 2003, 22,936 PHCs have been established against the total requirement of 23,000. Suggested norms of Health Manpower is as follows.

- Doctor : 1 per 3,500 population
- Nurse : 1 per 5,000 population
- Health worker (F & M) : 1 per 5,000 and 1 per 3,000 population
- Trained Dai : 1 per 1,000 population
- Health Assistant (M & F) : 1 per 30,000 and 1 per 20,000 Population
- Pharmacist : 1 per 10,000 population
- Laboratory Technician : 1 per 10,000 population

At present India has 56 doctors per 1,00,000 population, 9.3 beds per 10,000 population and 78 nurses and midwives per 1,00,000 population. These figures vary widely within the country. There is also mal-distribution of health manpower between rural and urban areas. The concentration of physician is much more in urban areas than in rural areas. This difference is attributed to absence of amenities in rural areas, lack of job satisfaction, equipmental insufficiency, professional isolation, lack of rural experience, inability to adjust to rural life and enormity of political disturbances.

In recent years there has been a change from unipurpose to multipurpose strategy. The WHO has set a goal of expenditure of 5% of each country's GNP on Health Care, while India is spending about 3% of GNP on Health and Family

Welfare programmes. In addition to finance, duty hours spent on actual health care is an important aspect. Administrative delays in sanctioning different health projects cause loss of time. Proper use of man-hours is another determining factor. The WHO in a survey on ANM has shown that an ANM on average spends 45% of her time in giving medical care, 40% in travelling, 5% in paper work and only 10% in performing duties for which she has been trained. Such studies if conducted on medical personnel may produce alarming results. In order to make the health services comprehensive, accessible, acceptable, providing scope for community participation and available at a cost that the community and country can afford, suitable strategies are to be introduced to get the optimum result.

Empowerment to Patients

To reduce the conflict in the field of health action, the patients (the health seekers) should also be active participants and should unconditionally have the power of decision-making. It is necessary to change the attitude on the part of health services providers so as to make the patients feel important, wanted, cared for and well looked after. This change in outlook must start early as part of the teaching curriculum, and should be the objectives for medical and paramedical students. They should realize that the hospitals of medical institutions need the patients for clinical teaching and thus the academia is dependent on the patients and not vice versa.

Usually, most of the patients seeking care in government hospitals are illiterate and ignorant of their rights. Due to lack of awareness the uninformed become passive consumers. To get these patients actively involved in their health management, they need to be awakened, informed, educated and enlightened to enable them to exercise their rights. Information would enable them to understand their health problems, know solutions through various options, understand the associated risks and anticipate solutions through the selected interventions. The patients own their bodies, associated illnesses and their values. It is their money that is involved in the public health systems. In many more ways they are the experts. Thus it is they who should have the power . . . It is their opinions that do matter. This part of education the patients should know.

PATIENTS AS DECISION-MAKERS

Informed and empowered patients can be dominant in decision-making in regard to choice of treatment intervention and choice of treatment with drug after knowing the possible adverse effects, addiction liability, cost-effectiveness, benefit-risk ratio and ultimate effect on their quality of life. In some clinical trials the empowered patients can volunteer to be part of research studies, drug trials or accept to be a case to be discussed with the medical students/faculties. From ethical point of view, they have every right to be informed and give consent before anaesthesia, surgery, invasive investigations, drug trials with known adverse effects. There should be some organization of empowered patients who can fight for restoring their rights, objection to strikes by doctors and nurses, banning the use of hazardous drugs and seeking rational drug treatment. The empowered patient group can influence a lot of decisions. The empowered patients can form a forum where they can get their complaints redressed with respect to negligence in daily routine, for example, laxity in nursing care, improper drug schedule. An efficient committee can be constituted with dedicated medical activists with representation from staff, medical social workers and individuals with keen interest in public health. The committee should work in informed style with ethical considerations and speed to satisfy the patients. This will save doctors and institutions from public interest litigations and consumer courts' intervention.

FEED-BACK FROM PATIENTS

Feed-back is an essential component of effective communication. Obtaining feed-back from empowered patients on an ongoing basis will help in evaluating success and utility of empowerment. This can be used to find shortcomings and a basis for further improvements in doctor-patient relationship.

BENEFITS OF EMPOWERMENT OF PATIENTS

Empowerment of patients will lead to medical uprising of the society by creating an educated and health-aware mass, informed and health conscious, striving to improve their quality of life through justified use of their rights. This can curb exploitation in the name of medicine and ensure a decline in quackery. The empowered can be easily motivated to give their support for health programmes and achievement of health goals. In this way the health programmes will be truly a people's programme. It will be easy to organize more patients and NGOs to protect long-term interests of patients. The health workers' approach will become more rational, self-regulatory, disciplined and patient-friendly. This will curb the malpractices in profession. It will give dignity of life to patients. Legal litigations and compensation suits will decrease. The patients will have more and more confidence in the health machinery. In the long run, the health status of empowered citizens will improve and will reduce the recurring expenditure in health management.

Doctor-Patient Relationship

By virtue of technical superiority, knowledge and skill, the doctor exercises an authoritative role and dominates the patient. The doctor must know how to communicate with his patient. Three levels of communication are necessary:

i. **Communication on an Emotional Plane:** The doctor should give a sympathetic and patient hearing to his patients and their relatives about their complaints. This will help establish a quick rapport and the patient will keep faith on his physician.

ii. **Communication on a Cultural Plane**: The physician must be familiar with the culture and social organization of the community. This will help him to acquire certain flexibility in his dealings with patients. The physician should give his scientific advice in terms of existing cultural pattern. Thus there will be a great chance that the doctor's advice will be totally followed by the patient.

iii. **Communication on an Intellectual Plane**: There is an enormous "social distance" between the physician and the patient. A successful doctor reduces this social distance and easily communicates with his patients freely and frankly and wins his confidence. One of the important components is the use of humour. It is the best ice breaker for the patient frozen by fear and anxiety.

A physician who is able to communicate with his patient on the above three planes can give maximum psychological satisfaction to his patients and help remove psychosomatic ailments. Patients are relieved of sorrow, miseries, fears, pain and agonies. This art has to be learnt by a successful physician for his and his patients' benefits, and ultimately the community and country will be benefited.

References

Dreze, Jean and Amartya Sen (1977), *India Economic Development and Social Opportunity*, Oxford University Press.

Park K. (2005), *Park's Text Book of Preventive and Social Medicine*, ed. 18, Jabalpur: M/s Banarasidas Bhanot.

Thawani, Vijay and Gharpure Kundu, (1997), *Health and Behaviour Empowering Patients*, Regional Health Forum, WHO, vol. 2, No. 1.

14

Some Feminist Concerns about Medical Practice

Shefali Moitra

THE gender question has been addressed by medical practitioners in a truncated way. First a division is made between general practitioners and gynaecologists. Consequently, it is claimed that the general practitioner is concerned with the neutered human body and the gynaecologist is concerned with the biological female. This division acknowledges the sex difference of females while it treats the male human subject as being representative of both males and females. Interestingly, when the aim is to show that women are not equal to men in physical strength and mental capabilities then the dimorphism between the sexes is accentuated. But when it comes to treatment of diseases then the difference in the chromosomal structure of men and women is ignored. A selective amnesia relating to identity or difference has far-reaching consequences for the doctor-patient relationship.

It is customary for biologists to commonly refer to primary, secondary and tertiary sex-linked characteristics. Chromosomes mark the primary sex-linked human traits while hormones characterize the secondary sex-linked characteristics. There is no qualitative difference between the hormones possessed by the males and those possessed by the females. Yet, their body chemistries differ due to the difference in chromosome structures. Neither the hormone secretion of all males is identical, nor the hormone secretion of all females is the same. The secondary sex-linked characteristics differ from individual to individual cutting across the primary male/female divide. The tertiary sex-linked characteristics are greatly influenced by the environment. By environment we mean both the natural and social environment. Tertiary sex-linked characteristics overlap gender.[1] The main difference between tertiary sex-linked characteristics and gender is that the former are treated as a biological category and the latter as a social category. The presence of a clear-cut black and white division between the biological and the social is being intensely debated.

There is a prevalent belief that by keeping the social and the biological domains separate, medicine can be approached in a more scientific manner. Throughout the history of modern medicine there has been a conscious effort to project medicine as a science and that too as a positivistic science. Physics is considered to be the model of positivistic science. Life sciences have always been looked upon by the physicist as a softer discipline. Perhaps this has been instrumental in pushing the medical sciences into a more defensive position.

By neutering human diseases like malaria, flu, small pox, etc. medical science takes on an objective approach to medicine. The point that medicine wants to establish is that it is unbiased, impersonal and invested in no particular point of view or not

---

1. Shefali Moitra, *Feminist Thought: Androcentrism, Communication and Objectivity*, Munshiram Manoharlal Publishers Pvt. Ltd., New Delhi, 2002, p. 7.

having a point of view. If medical practice deviates from this neutral position then that is a sign of malpractice and not an indication of inherent subjectivity in the medical sciences. Feminists argue that any neutral position taken either by medical science, or by the medical practitioner is an artificial position. In this way the whole picture is distorted. The science of medicine and the social underpinnings of medicine go hand in hand not only at the level of theory and practice but also at the level of medical data collection. We have already referred to tertiary sex-linked characteristics. They are a mixture of chromosomal structures, hormonal inputs and social influences; obviously these data need to be treated as being socially mediated and not as corporeal facts.

By treating diseases as human ailments of a generic type without having any relation to the sex/gender differences of an individual, great injustice is being done to woman's lived-experience. While preparing taxonomy of diseases and their symptoms the general practice is to use the male body as the model and the male experience as the source of symptomatic evidence. An investigation of the female body *vis-à-vis* generic diseases is either ignored or trivialized. The tradition of treating the male member of the human species as the representative individual is a consequence of patriarchy. In patriarchy males are foregrounded and females are back-grounded. It is presumed that other than having specific reproductive functions women are identical to men as far as generic diseases are concerned. In other words one section of medical science is concerned with the specific study of women's reproductive functions and their malfunctioning, and all other women-related complaints are relegated to general medicine.

J. Gittelsohn, P.J. Pelts, M.E. Bentley, M. Nag and N. Oomman[2] rightly point out, "Women's health is probably one of the most inadequately researched areas in international public health. A major flaw in past efforts has been an almost exclusive focus on women as mothers and child-care givers, rather than women themselves as a target population of interest." These researchers further observe that investigations into the cause of death of women in South Asia have been almost exclusively focused on deaths related to pregnancy and child delivery. From the statistics available one would then erroneously conclude that all the missing women referred to by Amartya Sen have gone missing on account of some reproductive health-related malady. Certainly this will be an oversimplification. What about the women who die due to injurious medical interventions aimed at making them more attractive models on the ramp? Where is the statistics on the cause of slow death of women who have to carry firewood and water on their heads or backs for miles? These are just a few examples of the kind of physical ailments to which women succumb. But what about the mental pressures that drive them to a pathological condition? Very little research is done to ascertain the gendered nature of these pathologies. Since patriarchy is concerned with the control of woman's productive and reproductive labour the patriarchal state and its medical institutions are not interested in the well-being of the post-menopausal woman. An enormous amount of money is put into Research and Development (R&D) relating to woman's reproductive health. The money put into R&D relating to post-menopausal health is only a small fraction of that.

---

2. J. Gittelsohn, et al., *Listening to Women Talking about their Health: Issues and Evidence from India*, 1994, p. 40.

The thrust of the kind of research work being done in relation to woman's reproductive health has little to do with women's reproductive rights. When it comes to birth control the entire onus is on the woman. Male contraceptives are not being aggressively marketed or prescribed as are female contraceptives. The availability of *de facto* reproductive rights is meagre in the Third World countries. Here the State and the family control woman's right to reproduction but at the same time no safe form of contraceptive has been offered for women. The Third World countries have become a safe dumping ground for unsafe contraceptive pills. In spite of the fact that there are clear instructions given with each phial of medicine that the drug should be administered only after certain tests are made on the patient, these precautions are openly flouted and the drugs are also available across the counter. There have been many street protests against the availability of these drugs, many letters have been written to the editors of leading newspapers but the result has been nil. Multiple vested interests are involved in these unethical transactions. These interests wield a significant amount of power.

When women fall ill they are commonly diagnosed to be suffering from some psychosomatic disorder meaning thereby that there is no real ailment; the ailment is there only in the mind. When it comes to identifying a syndrome women are commonly labelled as being hysteric. The word "hysteric" is derived from the Greek word *husterikos* meaning the womb (*hustera*). To be hysterical means to be morbidly or uncontrollably emotional. Hysteria is thought to occur more frequently in women than in men. This may be true but then why is it so? It is generally noticed that women feel more comfortable with their emotions than men do. Men try to deny their emotions. Not having emotions is often seen to be a manly virtue. Even when men feel emotions they are trained not to express them. Women on the other hand do not feel any social pressure to control their emotions. It is socially acceptable for a woman to express her pain in public whereas it is a taboo for men to do so. Apart from the different forms of social conditioning there is a deeper question involved here, "What makes women morbidly emotional?"

One of the major reasons for this morbidity is that adequate attention is not paid to their physical and mental well-being. By not acknowledging the specificities of their lived-experience medical practice glosses over a woman's lived-experience. This is not to say that women are not allowed a separate category; they are. The category imposed on them is the category of the feminine "other" of patriarchy. The sedimentation of cultural structures is largely responsible for this. The sedimentation of culture is so extensive and penetrating that it affects the mindset of both men and women. The invisibility of women's lived experience is not only the perception of men, it is also the perception of women. Women internalize the mindset of patriarchy to the extent that they begin to believe that man is the representative individual and woman is seen as a lack.

The deplorable state of women's health, especially in the Third World countries, is not only due to the negligence of the state and the family. Women themselves are also responsible for this sorry state of affairs. Most women nurture a very low self-image about their status and health rights; they neglect their health needs too. When a woman is oblivious of her worth she will automatically lose her desire to keep fit and healthy. Further, if her gender role is constructed in such a way that she is shrouded in mystery then the signifiers of her physical and mental state need also to be kept invisible. The Mona Lisa smile must be adorned to keep people guessing what the real message is. Under these circumstances the doctor may also get confused. The best way out of this dilemma for the doctor would be to fall back on his repertoire of stereotypical information gained from his study of the positivistic science of medicine. This falling back on stereotypes ignores the fact that historically women's lives have had dimensions different from men's.

The method of diagnosis needs to be re-examined under the circumstances of mystification of women in patriarchy. Part of the mystification process is closely related to a subsidiary practice of attributing a degree of divinity and magnanimity to women. Women are first and foremost seen as mothers. As mothers they are expected to be caring, nurturing and willing to sacrifice themselves for their children and family. They are referred to as homemakers. Cooking, cleaning, nursing are supposed to be the natural dispositions of women. Those who are efficient at performing these chores are eulogized as the goddess Lakshmi, the deity of wealth and prosperity. If one has to sacrifice one's health to earn this sobriquet then be it so. To perform like a goddess is not a sufficient condition for acquiring such recognition, one must also have the requisite features and appearance of a goddess, fair complexion, luscious hair and the proper vital statistics. To attain these standards women have to practise many regimens; many of these are detrimental to her health. Women are not only expected to mould their outward appearance according to certain given stereotypes, their attitude and disposition also need to be severely regimented. The physical prescriptions for being divine have far-reaching consequences on woman's health, including her mental health, and conversely the mental inhibitions and controls affect a woman's physical health. No wonder women are prone to hysterical outbursts, to morbidly uncontrollable emotions.

The presence of the feminine mystique may puzzle the medical practitioner. Seen in isolation the meaning of a feminine mystique cannot be decoded. Various social processes are involved here. These processes jointly produce a syndrome that has to be understood holistically. Issues of class, ethnicity, and religion join gender in many unanticipated ways. Unfortunately the psycho-social aspects of ailments have so far been taken up from a patriarchal point of view. It must be remembered that the doctor in a patriarchal set-up is a powerfully placed and institutionally accredited expert. Feminists who are contesting the authority of the doctor are looking at the relation of the models pursued by medical practice and socio-political ideologies. Many of the existing relationships need to be challenged.

When it comes to the diagnosis of women's ailments physicians have a tendency to "look through" and not "look at" the symptoms of the patient. The distinction between "looking through" and "looking at" is made by Richard Lanham in his *The Electronic Word: Democracy, Technology and the Arts* (1993).[3] While looking through the patient it is easy for the doctor to project his interpretation on to the patient. Since the doctor has the licence to knowledge he knows best. He is the one who can unilaterally decide whether the female patient's outburst is a case of hysteria, therefore pathology, or whether it is a normal reaction. The process of looking through allows the doctor to trivialize the patient's complaints, or to ignore their reporting; thus women are denied authority

---

3. Richard Lanham in *The Electronic Word: Democracy, Technology and the Arts*, Chicago University Press, Chicago, 1993, p. 5.

over their bodies. They are denied the right to semantic authorship. The doctor alone has the right to classify. Diana Long rightly observes, "We cannot leave it to the experts to tell us the proper names of our bodies or ourselves."[4]

By now it should be abundantly clear that a positivistic approach to medicine will not reveal the real existing state of affairs. Woman's body and its ailments are not lying out there as an objective reality waiting to be recognized. The meaning of the body and its parts and functions are one and all subjected to multiple meanings projected by society. In this entire game woman's voice is hardly heard and her agency seldom recognized. Wendy Harcourt rightly points out that the body is inherently part of social and political participation.[5] Harcourt says, "In this sense there is no neat divide between the corporeal and the social; the body is understood as a political site or place that mediates the lived experiences of social and cultural relationships."[6]

The international women's movement is acutely aware of the existing politics that is being played with women's bodies. Such awareness has led to a major shift in the area of population and development. The International Conference on Population and Development, held in Cairo in September 1994 shifted the focus of population programmes to the rights of women.

---

4. Diana Long, "Hidden Persuaders: Medical Indexing and the gendered Professionalism of American Medicine, 1880-1932" in *Women Gender and Science: New Directions,* Edited by Sally Gregory Kohlstedt and Helen Longino, *Osiris,* Second Series, Volume 12, 1997, p. 119.
5. Wendy Harcourt, "Body Politics: Revisiting the Population Question" in *Feminist Post-Development Thought,* edited by Kriemild Saunders, Zed Books, London, 2002, p. 293.
6. Wendy Harcourt, p. 292.

This shift was of partial help for the empowerment of women. The acknowledgement of rights over one's body within an overarching patriarchal system may not yield the desired empowerment. Patriarchal institutions and patriarchal practices also need to be critiqued. Medical science and medical practice is a major stake holder in the perpetuation of the patriarchal status quo. The United Nations Family Planning Association (UNFPA) website states, "at Cairo 179 countries agreed that population and development are inextricably linked, and that empowering women and meeting people's needs for education and health, including reproductive health are necessary for both individual advancement and balanced development." It is to be noted that improvement of health is not only to the benefit of the individual, it is beneficial for development in general. Secondly, it is also to be noted that health is coupled with education in bringing about development. The mere expansion of education will not bring about gender equality. An education system that critiques patriarchy needs to be introduced.

In order to bring about a change in the status of women and health care we need to have a proper data base. In this case merely a quantitative data base will not suffice. What is needed is a qualitative methodological approach. In the absence of such an investigation we will not be able to know the belief world of the patient nor will we be able to know the power structure of multinational pharmaceutical companies and the way they influence a doctor's decision. The mechanisms of various types of control, including state control need also to be exposed. The qualitative method of investigation is not opposed to the quantitative method; one can complement the other. The uniqueness of qualitative investigation is that it looks at various types of data that cannot be clearly quantified.

Contributors

Amit Kumar Sharma, Research Scholar, Department of Philosophy, Punjab University, Chandigarh.

Anup Kumar Dhar, Research Scholar, Asiatic Society, Kolkata.

Bansi Badan Mukhopadhyay, Associate Professor, Department of Community Medicine, Burdwan Medical College, Burdwan, West Bengal.

Chanda Gupta, Professor, Department of Philosophy, Jadav-pur University, Kolkata.

Debashis Chatterjee, Psychiatrist, Mon Foundation, Kolkata.

Gopaldeb Chattopadhyay, Assistant Director, Bureau of Applied Economics and Statistics, Burdwan, West Bengal.

Malay Kumar Basu, Formerl Judge, Kolkata High Court, Kolkata.

Nandini Banerjee, Registrar, Respiratory Medicine, Good Hope Hospital, NHS Trust, West Midlands, UK.

Pushpa Mishra, Formerly Principal, Bethune College, Kolkata.

Ranjita Biswas, Psychiatrist, Antara Gram Psychiatric Centre, Kolkata.

Ratna Dutta Sharma, Professor, Department of Philosophy, Jadavpur University, Kolkata.

S.Y. Khan, Consulting Physician, SSKM Hospital, Kolkata.

Sashinungla, Reader, Department of Philosophy, Jadavpur University, Kolkata.

Shefali Moitra, Professor, Department of Philosophy, Jadavpur University, Kolkata.

Somdatta Bhattacharyya, Lecturer, Department of Philosophy, P.D. Women's college, Jalpaiguri, West Bengal.

Swaraj Mazumdar, Consulting Homoeopath, Kolkata.

Index